Skills Practice Manual
for LaFleur Brooks'

HEALTH UNIT
Coordinating

Skills Practice Manual
for LaFleur Brooks'

HEALTH UNIT
Coordinating

SEVENTH EDITION

Elaine A. Gillingham, AAS, BA, CHUC
Program Director 1993 – 2005 (retired),
Health Unit Coordinating Program,
GateWay Community College,
Phoenix, Arizona

Monica Melzer Wadsworth Seibel, BS, MEd, CHUC
Program Director,
Health Unit Coordinating Program,
GateWay Community College,
Phoenix, Arizona

ELSEVIER

3251 Riverport Lane
St. Louis, Missouri 63043

Notices

Knowledge and best practice in this field are constantly changing. As new research and experience
broaden our understanding, changes in research methods, professional practices, or medical treatment may become necessary.

Practitioners and researchers must always rely on their own experience and knowledge in evalu-
ating and using any information, methods, compounds, or experiments described herein. In using
such information or methods they should be mindful of their own safety and the safety of others,
including parties for whom they have a professional responsibility.

With respect to any drug or pharmaceutical products identified, readers are advised to check the
most current information provided (i) on procedures featured or (ii) by the manufacturer of each
product to be administered, to verify the recommended dose or formula, the method and duration
of administration, and contraindications. It is the responsibility of practitioners, relying on their own
experience and knowledge of their patients, to make diagnoses, to determine dosages and the best
treatment for each individual patient, and to take all appropriate safety precautions.

To the fullest extent of the law, neither the Publisher nor the authors, contributors, or editors,
assume any liability for any injury and/or damage to persons or property as a matter of products liability, negligence or otherwise, or from any use or operation of any methods, products, instructions,
or ideas contained in the material herein.

Vice President and Publisher: Andrew Allen
Content Manager: Ellen Wurm-Cutter
Publishing Services Manager: Julie Eddy, Hemamalini Rajendrababu
Senior Project Manager: Celeste Clingan
Project Manager: Anitha Sivaraj
Design Direction: Karen Pauls

Printed in the United States of America

Last digit is the print number: 9   8   7   6   5   4   3

Preface

The 7th edition of *Skills Practice Manual for LaFleur Brooks' Health Unit Coordinating* reflects and corresponds with the latest changes made in *LaFleur Brooks' Health Unit Coordinating*, 7th edition. This edition also includes an online Practice Activity Software for Transcription of Physicians' Orders (see inside front cover for access instructions). The *LaFleur Brooks' Health Unit Coordinating* text provides the theory needed to perform the health unit coordinating job, and the skills manual and online resource provide hands-on practice in performing the transcription of doctors' orders and other tasks performed by the Health Unit Coordinator. Many hospitals have implemented the electronic medical record with computer physician order entry, which creates changes in the Health Unit Coordinator's role. See Chapter 1 in *LaFleur Brooks' Health Unit Coordinating*, 7th edition, for more information.

Chapter Design

The chapters correspond with the chapters of *LaFleur Brooks' Health Unit Coordinating*, 7th edition. The student learns the theory by reading the chapter, completing the exercises, reviewing questions in the text, and then practicing the task in this manual. Each activity begins with a list of materials needed and step-by-step instructions to complete the activity. Activities provided in Chapters 10 through 19 may be completed by using the online Practice Activity Software for Transcription of Physicians' Orders on a computer. When a computer is not available, the activities may be completed by using the sample downtime requisitions provided in Appendix B in the back of this manual. The sample requisitions contain information that is included in the online Practice Activity Software for Transcription of Physicians' Orders and would also be seen when transcribing doctors' orders using a hospital computer program. Handwritten doctors' orders are included in Appendix A for additional practice in transcription as well as reading handwriting

Online Practice Activity Resource

The online Practice Activity Software for Transcription of Physicians' Orders included in this manual simulates a hospital computer system that students may use for practice when transcribing the printed and handwritten doctors' orders provided. Options provided on the website for practice include the following:

- Enter orders.
- Print a nursing unit census.
- Admit a patient.
- Transfer a patient.
- Discharge a patient.
- Research location of patients admitted to the hospital by using "patient inquiry."
- Verify tests ordered by using "order inquiry."
- Cancel an order that has been entered.
- Research diagnostic test results by using "laboratory results" or "diagnostic imaging results."
- Locate or create a patient profile.
- Enter medications on a patient medication profile.
- Locate a doctor on the doctor's roster.

Patient forms may be printed from the website, making it possible for the student to practice the transcription process at home.

Clinical Evaluation Record

A clinical (on-the-job) evaluation is included in Appendix C of this manual to measure and record the student's performance on the nursing unit. It is divided into seven units; the first six are sequenced according to the increasing degree of knowledge and skill that the student needs to complete the unit. The objectives and corresponding activities will assist the student in mastering each of the tasks required. A rating scale is provided to measure and record the student's performance level.

The Clinical Evaluation Record tells the student, the instructor, and the preceptor exactly what is expected of the student during the student's clinical experience. Use of this record allows the student to pursue mastery of skills and to arrange an evaluation of skills by the instructor or preceptor. The completed appendix becomes a written record of the student's performance in the clinical setting. The appendix may be used by the instructor to assign grades or by the student to obtain employment. As does the rest of this manual, this appendix corresponds with the textbook *LaFleur Brooks' Health Unit Coordinating*, 7th edition.

Instructions to the Student

How To Use This Manual

This manual consists of 91 activities that provide practice for the health unit coordinator student to master skills in a simulated hospital setting (using paper charts) prior to actual hospital practice. It also includes a clinical evaluation record designed to measure and record the student's on-the-job performance.

The activities in this manual correspond to the content of the same-numbered chapters in the textbook *LaFleur Brooks' Health Unit Coordinating,* 7th edition. For best results, read each chapter and complete the exercises and review questions provided in each chapter of *LaFleur Brooks' Health Unit Coordinating* prior to performing the activities in this manual.

Chapters

The chapters are numbered and titled to correspond with the chapters of the textbook *LaFleur Brooks' Health Unit Coordinating,* 7th edition. The activities match the theory content of each chapter. Textbook chapters that do not require practice are not included in the manual. There are no activities included for Chapters 1, 2, 3, 5, 6, 9, 21, and 22.

Each chapter specifies the skill to be practiced, the materials needed to practice the skill, and the steps necessary to perform the skill, with check boxes provided to record completion of each step and of the whole activity. As each activity is completed (preferably after having been repeated until complete accuracy is achieved), either the instructor or the student should write a check in the completion box.

Chapters 4, 7, and 8 include practice in communication skills and in preparing and working with the patients' charts. Chapter 7 includes instruction and practice in preparing a census worksheet (may be printed from website), and Chapter 8 includes instruction and practice in assembling a patient's chart and charting of vital signs (forms may be printed from the website).

Chapters 10 through 18 provide practice in transcribing the different categories of doctors' orders. The steps of transcription are repeated in each activity to provide the student with an orderly learning experience and a useful summary for future reference.

Chapters 19 and 20 provide practice in performing health unit coordinating tasks, such as admission, preoperative and postoperative procedures, and discharge orders.

Supplies Needed by the Student include the following:
- Computer (when available)
- Black ink pen
- Red ink pen
- Pencil
- Eraser
- Yellow highlighter

Check with your instructor for additional required supplies.

Suggestions to the Student for Maximum Use of Chapters 10 Through 18

1. At the beginning of each activity, steps may be deleted or added to adapt the procedure to the practice in your area.
2. Record in the following spaces the symbols used to indicate completion of the transcription steps:
   _____ Kardexing
   _____ Ordering (either by computer or requisition)
   _____ Recording the medication on the medication administration record
   _____ Completing a telephone call
   _____ Faxing or sending the pharmacy copy of the physicians' order sheet
3. Record the colors of ink to be used for the transcription process.
4. Remove all physicians' orders provided in the activities as directed and place them in the chart binder that you prepared in Chapter 8 to simulate hospital practice.
5. Generic forms and examples of downtime requisitions that may be used when computers are not available are provided in Appendix B. You may duplicate these or use forms and requisitions supplied by your instructor to complete the activities.
6. To practice transcribing orders by the computer method, simply use the computer to perform the ordering step by following the instructions included in each activity and the Practice Activity Software for Transcription of Physicians' Orders.
7. Fill in today's date, time, and doctors' names on each practice doctors' order sheet prior to starting the transcription process.
8. Hospitals using paper charts require that the physicians' orders be faxed to the pharmacy or the pharmacy copy sent. This activity may not be practiced in the classroom.

Appendix A

Appendix A consists of sets of actual doctors' orders. They contain many orders not included in the activities and are written as they might be seen in the actual hospital environment. The sets of orders provide experience in automatic cancellation, renewals, and changes. Practice transcribing the sets of doctors' orders by the computer method using the Practice Activity Software for Transcription of Physicians' Orders or the requisition method by using the requisitions provided and the 10 steps of transcription.

Appendix B

Generic downtime requisitions that may be used (when computers are not available) as necessary to complete the activities are included in Appendix B. Reproduce as many of each as are needed for each activity.

Appendix C

Appendix C is a Clinical Evaluation Record, designed to measure and record the student's performance in the hospital setting. A rating scale is included to measure and record the student's level of performance. The student should take the Clinical Evaluation Record to the hospital site each day and use it as a guide in obtaining on-the-job experiences and an evaluation rating from his or her preceptor or instructor.

Many of the skills included in this Clinical Evaluation Record are critical; that is, an error in performing them on the job could cause harm to the patient. We hope that by working your way through the activities, you will become both competent and confident in your practice, and that you will be ready to accept the full responsibilities of a career in Health Unit Coordinating.

Contents

CHAPTER 4

Communication Devices and Their Uses

Activities in this Chapter:

4–1: Answer the Telephone
4–2: Place a Telephone Caller on Hold
4–3: Transcribe a Telephone Message
4–4: Place a Telephone Call to a Doctor's Office
4–5: Leave a Voice Mail Message
4–6: Contact a Person Using a Digital Pager

★ HIGH PRIORITY

Telephone techniques and use of other communication devices may be reviewed in Chapter 4 of *LaFleur Brooks' Health Unit Coordinating*, 7th edition.

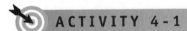 **ACTIVITY 4-1**

ANSWER THE TELEPHONE

Materials Needed   Telephone

Situation

You are a student health unit coordinator (HUC) working on an orthopedic unit, 3 East, at Opportunity Medical Center.

Directions

Practice answering the telephone using the information provided. Perform the following steps. Place a check mark (✓) in the box as you complete each step.

1

Steps for Answering the Telephone

1. Answer the telephone promptly (preferably before third ring).   ☐

2. Identify:
   a. the nursing unit   ☐
   b. yourself (give your first name)   ☐
   c. your status   ☐

3. Follow correct telephone etiquette by:
   a. speaking into the telephone mouthpiece   ☐
   b. giving the caller your undivided attention   ☐
   c. being courteous at all times   ☐
   d. speaking distinctly and clearly   ☐

Place a check mark (✔) in the following box to indicate that you have completed Activity 4-1.

☐ Answer the Telephone   Date: _____

🎯 **ACTIVITY 4-2**

PLACE A TELEPHONE CALLER ON HOLD

Materials Needed   Telephone
                          Pen or pencil
                          Note pad

Situation

You receive a telephone call from Dr. Robert Cohen requesting to speak to Joan, the case manager for Mary Sanchez regarding discharging Mary to Bryant's Rehab Center.

Directions

Practice placing a telephone caller on hold using the information provided. Perform the following steps. Place a check mark (✔) in the box as you complete each step.

Steps for Placing a Telephone Caller on Hold

1. Follow the steps for answering the telephone as directed in Activity 4-1.   ☐

2. Write the name of the caller, the nature of the call, and the appropriate telephone line on a note pad.   ☐

NOTE PAD

Name of the caller: _____

Telephone line number: _____

Message: _____

_____

---

3. Ask for permission to place the caller on hold (using appropriate telephone etiquette); wait for an answer. ❑

4. Press the *hold* button. ❑

5. Notify Joan, the case manager, of the call and the information, including the telephone line of the call. ❑

Place a check mark (✓) in the following box to indicate that you have completed Activity 4–2.

❑ Place a Telephone Caller on Hold   Date: _____

★ HIGH PRIORITY

Always return to the person on hold every 30 to 60 seconds to ask if they wish to remain on hold or leave a number for a return call.

★ HIGH PRIORITY

If an electronic medical record (EMR) system is used, Dr. Cohen may enter a message for Joan, the case manager, into Mary's EMR, or if wireless devices (such as a Vocera) are in use, Dr. Cohen may call Joan directly.

⊙ ACTIVITY 4 - 3

TRANSCRIBE A TELEPHONE MESSAGE

Materials Needed   Telephone
                       Pen or pencil
                       Note pad

Situation

A telephone call is received from Dr. Olivia Petein providing the following directions: "Notify Paul Mosher's nurse that I will be there within an hour to perform an LP and that I'll need an LP tray, liquid Betadine, and size 8½ gloves at the bedside."

Directions

Practice transcribing a telephone message using the information provided. Perform the following steps. Place a check mark (✓) in the box as you complete each step.

Steps for Transcribing a Telephone Message

1. Follow the steps for answering the telephone as directed in Activity 4-1.   ☐

2. Write the following information from the message on a note pad: ☐

NOTE PAD

The person's name for whom the message is intended: _____

The caller's name: _____

The date and time of the call: _____

_____

The message: _____

_____

_____

_____

The telephone number of the caller if a return call is expected: _____

Sign with your first and last name: _____

★ HIGH PRIORITY

If an EMR system is used, Dr. Petein may enter a message for Paul's nurse, or if wireless devices (such as a Vocera) are in use, Dr. Petein may call Paul's nurse directly.

Place a check mark (✔) in the following box to indicate that you have completed Activity 4-3.

☐ Transcribe a Telephone Message   Date: _____

◎ ACTIVITY 4-4

PLACE A TELEPHONE CALL TO A DOCTOR'S OFFICE

Materials Needed   Telephone

Pen or pencil

Note pad

Simulated doctors' roster provided by your instructor

or

Computer with Practice Activity Software for Transcription of Physicians' Orders (simulated doctors' roster)

Situation

Ted Pollack, one of the registered nurses (RNs) on the unit, requests that a call be placed to Jesus Mendez's doctor, Dr. John Seeley, to obtain an order for an antiemetic for Jesus's nausea and vomiting.

Directions

Practice placing a telephone call to a doctor's office using the information provided previously. Perform the following steps. Place a check mark (✓) in the box as you complete each step.

Steps for Placing a Telephone Call to a Doctor's Office

1. Plan the call by writing the following information on a note pad: ❑

NOTE PAD

The patient's name: _____

The telephone number of the doctor's office (this will save time if the telephone line is

busy or you have to return the call): _____

The reason for the call: _____

The person requesting the call: _____

The time the call is placed: _____

The name of the person spoken to: _____

---

2. Obtain the patient's chart. ❑

3. Select the correct physician using the doctors' roster provided by your instructor or the simulated doctors' roster from the Practice Activity Software by referring to:
  a. the first and last name of the physician ❑
  b. the specialty area ❑

4. Place the call to the doctor's office. ❑

5. Follow the telephone etiquette outlined in Activity 4-1. ❑

6. Give the following information when the telephone is answered:
  a. your name ❑
  b. your status ❑
  c. the name of the hospital ❑
  d. the name of the nursing unit ❑
  e. a return telephone number ❑
  f. the relevant information written in step 1 ❑

SCENARIO

"This is Sandy, the HUC on 3 East at Opportunity Medical Center. Jesus Mendez's nurse, Ted, would like to speak to Dr. Seeley regarding an antiemetic order for Mr. Mendez to relieve his nausea and vomiting."

---

7. Write the time of call and the name of the person you spoke to on the note pad. ❑

8. Notify Ted Pollack that the call has been placed. ❑

★ HIGH PRIORITY

When wireless devices such as Voceras are used, Ted may call Dr. Seely directly to obtain an order for an antiemetic.

Place a check mark (✔) in the following box to indicate that you have completed Activity 4-4.

☐ Place a Telephone Call to a Doctor's Office   Date: _____

🎯 ACTIVITY 4-5

LEAVE A VOICE MAIL MESSAGE

Materials Needed   Telephone
Recorder

Situation

The nurse manager, Paula Clarkson, has requested that you call Keith Jackson and leave a voice mail message letting him know that his assigned shift tonight is cancelled and that he should call her in the morning.

Directions

Practice leaving a voice mail message on a recorder using the previous information. Perform the following steps. Place a check mark (✔) in the box as you complete each step.

Steps for Leaving a Voice Mail Message

1. Dial the telephone number supplied to you by your instructor.   ☐

2. After listening to the recorded greeting and indicated tone, say your name, hospital name, the nursing unit, the time, and the message. Be sure to speak slowly and distinctly.   ☐

3. State the nurse manager's name and telephone number during the message and repeat the name and number at the end of the message.   ☐

Place a check mark (✔) in the following box to indicate that you have completed Activity 4-5.

☐ Leave a Voice Mail Message   Date: _____

🎯 ACTIVITY 4-6

CONTACT A PERSON USING A DIGITAL PAGER

Materials Needed   Digital pager
Telephone
List of pager numbers
Note pad

Situation

Cindy, an RN, requests that you page the hospitalist regarding her patient's (Ellen Graves) blood sugar test results.

Directions

Practice contacting a person using a digital pager. Perform the following steps. Place a check mark (✓) in the box as you complete each step.

Steps for Contacting a Person Using a Digital Pager

1. Write the following information on a note pad: ❑

NOTE PAD

The name of the person to be paged: _____

The pager number: _____

The return telephone number: _____

The time of the page: _____

Note: It may be necessary to obtain an outside line when paging a person outside the hospital before proceeding with the remaining steps.

2. Dial the pager number from a touch-tone telephone. ❑

3. Listen for a ring followed by a series of beeps. ❑

4. Enter the return telephone number followed by the pound sign (#) to display the number on the pager. ❑

Note: Some hospitals use a code number indicating urgency for return call (1 = stat, 2 = ASAP) that is entered after the return number.

5. Listen for a series of beeps or a "thank you" message, which indicates the page was completed. ❑

Place a check mark (✔) in the following box to indicate that you have completed Activity 4-6.

❑ Contact a Person Using a Digital Pager   Date: _____

⭐ **HIGH PRIORITY**

When wireless devices (such as a Vocera) are used, Cindy and the hospitalist may speak directly.

CHAPTER 7

Management Techniques and Problem-Solving Skills for Health Unit Coordinating

Activities in this Chapter:

7–1: Prepare a Unit Census Worksheet

> ★ **HIGH PRIORITY**
>
> Information regarding a unit census worksheet or patient activity sheet may be reviewed in Chapter 7 of *LaFleur Brooks' Health Unit Coordinating*, 7th edition.

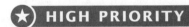 **ACTIVITY 7-1**

PREPARE A UNIT CENSUS WORKSHEET

Materials Needed

Pen or pencil

Patient activity sheet from Appendix B in this book

or

Computer with Practice Activity Software for Transcription of Physicians' Orders located on the Evolve web site

Situation

You are the health unit coordinator (HUC) on the morning shift for a surgical unit at Opportunity Medical Center. Nancy Clary, registered nurse, has left the following tape-recorded change-of-shift report at the end of her night shift.

> ★ **HIGH PRIORITY**
>
> An HUC may listen to the nurse's report or may receive a report from the HUC going off duty.

Change-of-Shift Report

Joseph Smith (room 401, bed 1) is a 42-year-old with a diagnosis of diabetes mellitus, admitted with gangrene of his right foot. He is scheduled for an amputation of his right leg up to the knee tomorrow morning. Joe had a good night, but is quite depressed. His blood sugar has been in the normal range, and he has had his 6:00 AM insulin this morning. Dr. Franks has requested that Joe's AM labs be called to his office today.

Anthony Garcia (room 401, bed 2) is a 20-year-old admitted with appendicitis at 3:00 AM this morning. He has signed his surgery consent and will be going to surgery to follow the 7:30 AM case. There is a pre-op order on call. He has slept off and on since admission, and his girlfriend will be back prior to his surgery. He seems to be a little apprehensive about going to surgery. This is his first hospital admission.

Sally Forest (room 402, bed 1) is a 28-year-old who was admitted 2 days ago after a motor vehicle accident. She had a concussion, fractured ribs, and minor cuts and bruises. She had a restful night, and Dr. Jones has written her discharge for this morning.

Tillie Frankel (room 402, bed 2) is a 70-year-old admitted last Thursday with a diagnosis of a cerebral vascular accident. Tillie is still on O_2 at 2 L/min per nasal prongs, has an IV of lactated Ringer's running, and had a pretty restless night. She had urinary incontinence twice during the night. She is afebrile. Her total intake during the night was 1450 mL with output approximately 800 mL. Physical therapy will be doing passive exercises this morning. Her husband stayed in her room last night and has requested that no other visitors be allowed.

★ HIGH PRIORITY

Each nurse going off duty will give a report (in person or tape recorded) about his or her assigned patients to the nurses coming on duty. Information will include the patient's name, room and bed number, age, diagnosis, reason for admission, date and type of surgery if applicable, significant changes in the patient's condition, results of tests and procedures during the last shift, tests and procedures scheduled for the upcoming shift, current physical and emotional assessments, vital signs if abnormal, intake and output, intravenous fluid status, activity, discharge planning, and an update on changes or effectiveness of care plan. The HUC will write down information that would be necessary to track the patients' conditions and activities. This will aid in performing required duties and tasks related to the patients.

Directions

Practice preparing a unit census worksheet using the information in the previous situation. Perform the following steps. Place a check mark (✓) in the box as you complete each step.

Steps for Preparing a Unit Census Sheet

1. Print a unit census worksheet from the Practice Activity Software for Transcription of Physicians' Orders located on the Evolve web site by choosing "census" from the home screen, and then choosing the worksheet tab (If not available, use the patient activity sheet from Appendix B in this book. Write out the room numbers and patients' names.)   ❑

2. Have someone read the change-of-shift report to you while you write pertinent information on the unit census worksheet or patient activity sheet.   ❑

3. Write the following information for each patient next to his or her name:
   a. any scheduled diagnostic procedure or surgery   ❑
   b. any planned discharge, transfer, or admission   ❑
   c. any do-not-resuscitate order   ❑
   d. whether visitors are allowed   ❑
   e. whether there is any do-not-release information   ❑
   f. any isolation procedures or infectious disease precautions.   ❑
   g. whether telephone calls are allowed   ❑
   h. any special reports that need to be placed in the chart   ❑
   i. any information, such as laboratory results, that needs to be called to a doctor's office when available   ❑

Place a check mark (✓) in the following box to indicate that you have completed Activity 7-1.

❑ Prepare a Unit Census Worksheet or Patient Activity Sheet   Date: _____

CHAPTER 8

The Patient's Chart

Activities in this Chapter

8-1: Convert Standard Time to Military Time and Military Time to Standard Time

8-2: Prepare a Patient's Chart

8-3: Document Vital Signs F (Fahrenheit Temperature) and Other Data on a Graphic Record

8-4: Document Vital Signs C (Celsius Temperature) and Other Data on a Graphic Record

8-5: Prepare a Consent Form

8-6: Correct a Labeling or Imprinter Error on a Chart Form

8-7: Correct a Written Error on a Chart Form

★ HIGH PRIORITY

When an electronic medical record (EMR) with computerized physician order entry system has been implemented, the patients' medical records will be computerized and there will be no need to assemble paper charts. Before the EMR system is implemented nationwide, you may be completing clinical experience and obtaining a job in which paper charts are used. The activities included in this chapter provide a foundation of knowledge of the forms used to document care and treatment, which will be valuable for using both paper charts and the EMR system.

★ HIGH PRIORITY

Military time, assembly of patients' charts, and the definitions and purposes of various chart forms may be reviewed in Chapter 8 of *LaFleur Brooks' Health Unit Coordinating*, 7th edition.

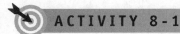 **ACTIVITY 8-1**

CONVERT STANDARD TIME TO MILITARY TIME AND MILITARY TIME TO STANDARD TIME

Materials Needed   Pen or pencil

Directions

Convert the listed standard times in the first column to military times. Convert the listed military times in the second column to standard times. Refer to the clock illustration as needed. Follow all steps. Place a check mark (✓) in the box as you complete each step.

Column 1

1. 12:00 pm   _12:00_
2. 1:15 pm   _13:15_
3. 6:27 pm   _18:27_
4. 4:13 pm   _16:13_
5. 7:05 pm   _19:05_
6. 1:35 pm   _13:35_
7. 11:30 pm   _23:30_
8. 2:00 pm   _14:00_
9. 8:25 pm   _20:25_
10. 5:15 pm   _17:15_

Column 2

1. 2400   _12 Am_
2. 2119   _9:19_
3. 0001   _12:01_
4. 0820   _8:20 Am_
5. 1919   _7:19 Pm_
6. 0605   _6:05 Am_
7. 2000   _8:00 Pm_
8. 0900   _9:00 Am_
9. 1200   _noon_
10. 1700   _4:00pm_

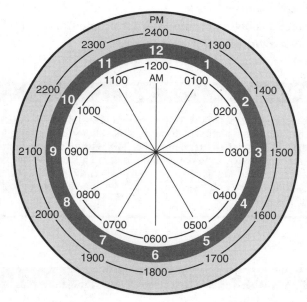

Steps for Converting Standard Time to Military Time and Military Time to Standard Time

1. Write the corresponding military time on the line next to the standard time in column 1:
   a. military times are written with four spaces (e.g., 9:00 AM = 0900; 12:00 noon = 1200) ☐
   b. spaces one and two designate the hour and spaces three and four designate the minutes (AM and PM are not used) ☐
   c. hours after midnight are 0100 to 1200 ☐
   d. a zero is used before the hours 1:00 AM through 9:00 AM to provide four spaces (0100 through 0900) ☐
   e. twelve noon is written as 1200 and the hours that follow are calculated by adding that number to 1200 (e.g., 6:00 PM is 600 + 1200 = 1800) up to midnight (2400) ☐

2. Write the corresponding standard time on the line next to military time in column 2:
   a. standard times use a colon and "AM" to designate hours between 12 midnight and 12 noon or "PM" to designate hours between 12 noon and 12 midnight
   b. twelve midnight is 12:00 AM and 12 noon is 12:00 PM
   c. hours between 12 midnight and 12 noon may be recognized by the "0" in the first space
   d. hours that follow 12 noon may be arrived at by subtracting 1200 (example: 1400 − 1200 = 200 = 2:00 PM)

★ HIGH PRIORITY

The use of military time eliminates confusion because hours are not repeated and the use of AM and PM is unnecessary.

Place a check mark (✓) in the following box to indicate that you have completed Activity 8-1.

☐ Convert Standard Time to Military Time and Military Time to Standard Time

Date: _____

◎ ACTIVITY 8-2

PREPARE A PATIENT'S CHART

Materials Needed

Pens

Patient ID labels

Chart binder and dividers

Patient chart forms listed in step 1

Patient profile printed from the Practice Activity Software located on the Evolve web site

Computer and Practice Activity Software for Transcription of Physicians' Orders located on the Evolve web site

Directions

Prepare a patient's chart by performing the following steps. Check with your instructor for variations of the procedure to adapt it to the practice in your area. Place a check mark (✓) in the box as you complete each step.

Steps for Preparing a Patient's Chart

1. Remove the following standard patient chart forms from Appendix B or print the forms from the Practice Activity Software located on the Evolve web site:
   a. Admission Service Agreement (Condition of Admission) form—initiated in the admitting department
   b. Information Sheet (Face Sheet or Patient Profile)—initiated in the admitting department
   c. Advance Directive Checklist—initiated in the admitting department
   d. Physicians' Order Sheet
   e. Physicians' Progress Record
   f. Nurses' Admission Record
   g. Nurses' Progress Notes (Nurses' Notes and Activity Flow Sheet)
   h. Graphic Record Form
   i. Medication Administration Record (MAR)
   j. Nurses' Discharge-Planning Form
   k. Physicians' Discharge Summary
   l. History and Physical Examination Form (this form may not be available until after the patient is admitted)

★ HIGH PRIORITY

Each patient must have an MAR that a registered nurse will sign at the end of each shift to indicate what medications the patient received or that the patient did not receive any medications during that shift.

★ HIGH PRIORITY

For future reference, make a list of any other standard chart forms used in your area.

2. Label each standard chart form with your patient's ID label. (If labels are not available, write the patient's information in black ink on each form.) You may choose a patient from the list of patients provided in the practice software or create your own patient by making up a name, an age, and the name of an admitting doctor. ☐

3. Fill in dates in ink where required on the forms. ☐

4. Label the chart binder with:
   a. the patient's name ☐
   b. the doctor's name ☐
   c. the room and bed number ☐

5. Place the completed standard patient chart forms in the patient's chart holder behind the correct divider. ☐

Place a check mark (✓) in the following box to indicate that you have completed Activity 8-2.

☐ Prepare a Patient's Chart   Date: _____

◎ ACTIVITY 8-3

DOCUMENT VITAL SIGNS F (FAHRENHEIT TEMPERATURE) AND OTHER DATA ON A GRAPHIC RECORD

Materials Needed   Black ink pen

Red ink pen (depending on hospital policy)

Labeled graphic record with headings (may be printed from Practice Activity Software for Transcription of Physicians' Orders located on the Evolve web site or may be copied from graphic forms included in Appendix B)

Directions

Practice documenting the vital signs and other data shown in the vital signs chart on the graphic record by following the steps below. Refer to Figure 8-1 for examples. Place a check mark (✓) in the box as you complete each step.

★ HIGH PRIORITY

Health care facilities and nursing units vary in distribution of responsibilities. Documenting vital signs may or may not be the responsibility of the HUC.

FIRST DAY

Time	T	P	R	BP	Stool	Wt
0800	100	104	18	136/92	÷	137
1200	100.2 Ⓡ	104	18			
1600	99.8	96	20	120/80	∴̈	
2000	102	80 ª	16			

SECOND DAY

Time	T	P	R	BP	Stool	Wt
0800	98.6 Ⓡ	84	22	120/100	·̈	140
1200	97.6	90 ª	16			
1600	98	80	18	132/90	∴̈	
2000	103.2 Ⓡ	60	16			

Figure 8.1

Steps to Documenting Vital Signs F (Fahrenheit Temperature) and Other Data on a Graphic Record

1. Document the Fahrenheit (F) temperature by:
   a. locating the matching temperature in the temperature column on the left side of the graphic record (Figure 8-2)

> ### ★ HIGH PRIORITY
>
> For the first temperature entry, circle the temperature number on the left side of the graphic record. Eventually the record may be microfilmed for storage; this step will indicate which graph line is a temperature.
> *Example:* The Fahrenheit temperature is 100.2°. Circle 100 in the temperature column.

   b. following the correct line to the right (each line is 0.2°) and stopping in the middle of the correct time column under the correct date
   c. placing a solid dot in ink on the line

> ### ★ HIGH PRIORITY
>
> Write an ® in ink above the dot to indicate a rectal temperature. Write an ˢA in ink above the dot to indicate an axillary temperature. For the first temperature entry, circle the temperature on the left side of the graphic record.
> *Example:* The temperature is 99° in the temperature column. Draw a line to the charted temperature. See the sample graphic record.

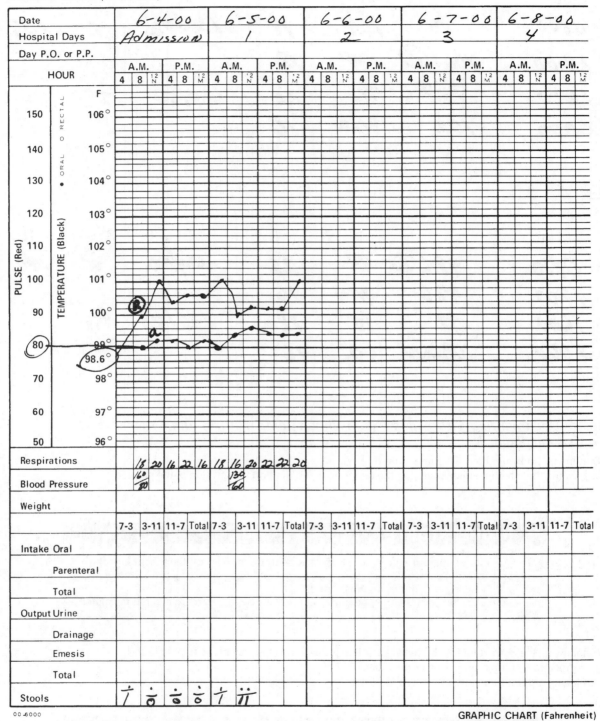

GRAPHIC CHART (Fahrenheit)

Figure 8.2

    d. connecting the dot in ink with the previous documented temperature, if the temperature is not a first entry   ❑

    e. drawing a line through the temperature in the vital signs chart (Figure 8-1) to indicate that it has been documented on the graphic record   ❑

2. Document the pulse by:

    a. locating the matching pulse in the pulse column on the left side of the graphic record   ❑

★ HIGH PRIORITY

For the first pulse entry, circle the pulse on the left side of the graphic chart. *Example:* The pulse is 102. Circle 100 in the pulse column. Draw a line to the charted pulse. See the sample graphic record.

---

    b. following the correct line to the right (each line is equal to two counts of a pulse) and stopping in the middle of the correct time column under the appropriate date   ❑

    c. placing a solid dot in ink on the line   ❑

★ HIGH PRIORITY

To indicate an apical pulse, write an "a" above the dot.

---

    d. connecting the dot in ink with the previous documented pulse, if the pulse is not a first entry   ❑

    e. drawing a line through the pulse in the vital signs chart to indicate that it has been documented on the graphic record   ❑

3. Document the respiratory rate by:

    a. locating the respiration heading on the left side of the graphic record   ❑

    b. following this row to the right and stopping at the correct time column under the appropriate date   ❑

    c. writing the respiratory rate in ink in the space   ❑

    e. drawing a line through the respiratory rate in the vital signs chart to indicate that it has been documented on the graphic record   ❑

4. Document the blood pressure by:

    a. locating the blood pressure heading on the left side of the graphic record   ❑

    b. following this row to the right and stopping at the correct time column under the appropriate date   ❑

    c. writing the blood pressure in ink in the space   ❑

    d. drawing a line through the blood pressure in the vital signs chart to indicate that it has been documented on the graphic record   ❑

5. Document the absence or number of stools by:

    a. locating the stool heading on the left side of the graphic chart   ❑

    b. following this row to the right and stopping in the correct time column under the appropriate date   ❑

    c. writing the symbol for the stools in ink in the space provided on the graphic record   ❑

Example:

No stools

One stool

Two stools

    d. drawing a line through the information on stools in the vital signs chart to indicate that it has been documented on the graphic chart   ❑

6. Document the weight by:

    a. locating the weight column on the left side of the graphic chart   ❑

    b. following this row to the right and stopping in the correct time column under the appropriate date   ❑

    c. writing the weight in ink in the space   ❑

    d. drawing a line through the weight in the vital signs chart to indicate that it has been documented on the graphic chart   ❑

7. Repeat each step as necessary to document the vital signs and other data for each time frame and date.   ❑

Place a check mark (✓) in the box below to indicate that you have completed Activity 8-3.

☐ Document Vital Signs F (Fahrenheit Temperature) and
Other Data on the Graphic Chart

Date: _____

 ACTIVITY 8-4

DOCUMENT VITAL SIGNS C (CELSIUS TEMPERATURE) AND OTHER DATA ON A GRAPHIC RECORD

Materials Needed   Black ink pen
Red ink pen (depending on hospital policy)
Labeled graphic record with headings

Directions

Practice documenting the vital signs and other data in shown in vital signs chart (Figure 8-3) on the graphic record by following the directions and steps in Activity 8-3.

> **★ HIGH PRIORITY**
>
> On the Celsius column of the graphic record, each line equals 0.1°.

FIRST DAY

Time	P	P	R	BP	Stool	Wt
8:00 A.M.	36.1	82	18	120/80	÷	188
12:00 Noon	37	102a	20			
4:00 P.M	32.5	98	16			
8:00 P.M.	38.2Ⓡ	80	20	120/80		

Second DAY

Time	T	P	R	BP	Stool	Wt
8:00 A.M.	37.1	88	16	140/100	⊤	190
12:00 Noon	34.4	100	20			
4:00 P.M.	36.5	66a	18			
8:00 P.M.	37Ⓐ	80	22	144/98	⁞⁄‖‖	

Figure 8.3

Place a check mark (✓) in the box below to indicate that you have completed Activity 8-4.

☐ Document Vital Signs C (Celsius Temperature)
and Other Data on a Graphic Record   Date: _____

◎ ACTIVITY 8-5

PREPARE A CONSENT FORM

Materials Needed   Patient ID labels
Consent form for surgery

Situation

A patient was admitted to the surgical unit at Opportunity Medical Center with a diagnosis of acute appendicitis. The patient's doctor writes an order for Dr. Peter Strauss to perform an appendectomy.

Directions

Practice preparing a consent form for surgery using the information provided previously. Perform the following steps. Check with your instructor for variations of the procedure to adapt it to the practice in your area. Place a check mark (✓) in the box as you complete each step.

Steps for Preparing a Consent Form for Surgery

1. Obtain a consent form for surgery from Appendix B of this book or from the practice activity software located on the Evolve web site.

2. Affix the patient's ID label on the consent form. (If labels are not available, write the patient's information on the consent form.)

3. Fill in the consent form in ink by writing:
a. the first and last name of the patient
b. the first and last name of the physician (note that the ordering physician is not the surgeon in this situation)
c. the surgery or procedure exactly as the doctor wrote it in their orders (do not abbreviate)

> ⭐ **HIGH PRIORITY**
>
> All written information must be spelled correctly and written legibly on consent forms. The nurse or physician will sign as a witness and write in the date and time after the patient has signed the consent.

4. Place the consent form in the chart binder for reference.

> ⭐ **HIGH PRIORITY**
>
> A consent form is also used for invasive medical procedures. Follow the same steps when filling out a consent form for a medical procedure.

> ⭐ **HIGH PRIORITY**
>
> Health care facilities have a policy that requires a licensed health care provider to witness the signing of a consent form. Telephone consents require two witnesses to listen to a verbal consent given over the telephone. Both will sign as witnesses on the consent form.

Place a check mark (✓) in the following box to indicate that you have completed Activity 8-5.

☐ Prepare a Consent Form   Date: _____

  ACTIVITY 8-6

CORRECT A LABELING OR IMPRINTER ERROR ON A CHART FORM

Materials Needed   Patient ID label
                        Physicians' order sheet

Situation

While you are checking your patient's chart, you discover that the doctor's order sheet was incorrectly given a different patient's label.

Directions

Practice correcting the labeling error on the following form using the information provided previously. Use the following steps. Check with your instructor for variations of the procedure to adapt it to the practice in your area. Place a check mark (✓) in the box as you complete each step.

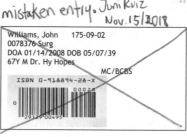
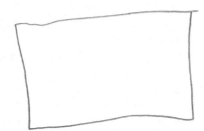

mistaken entry. Juni Ruiz Nov.15/2018

Williams, John   175-09-02
0078376 Surg
DOA 01/14/2008 DOB 05/07/39
67Y M Dr. Hy Hopes
                    MC/BCBS
ISBN 0-918894-28-X

PHYSICIANS' ORDER SHEET

Date	Time	Symbol	Orders

Steps for Correcting a Labeling or Imprinter Error on a Chart Form

1. Place the correct patient ID label, or write the correct information in ink, next to the error. ☐
2. Write an "X" in ink through the incorrect information (label). ☐
3. Write the words "mistaken entry" in ink above the error. ☐
4. Write the date, time, your first initial, your last name, and your status next to the words "mistaken entry." ☐

★ High Priority

Following proper procedure to correct an error on the patient's chart is important because the chart is a legal document and may be used as evidence in a court of law.

Place a check mark (✓) in the following box to indicate that you have completed Activity 8-6.

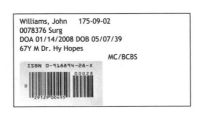

★ **HIGH PRIORITY**

Do not simply place the correct patient ID label over the incorrect label. The correct label could be removed or fall off the form.

☐ Correct a Labeling or Imprinter Error on a Chart Form   Date: _____

◉ **ACTIVITY 8-7**

CORRECT A WRITTEN ERROR ON A CHART FORM

Materials Needed   Black ink pen

Situation

The physician writes an order for hydroxyzine 25 mg PO prn for itching. The order is mistakenly written on the MAR as "hydralazine."

Directions

Practice correcting a written error on the MAR below, using the information provided previously. Perform the following steps. Check with your instructor for variations of the procedure to adapt it to the practice in your area. Place a check mark (✓) in the box as you complete each step.

```
Williams, John    175-09-02
0078376 Surg
DOA 01/14/2008 DOB 05/07/39
67Y M Dr. Hy Hopes
                        MC/BCBS

ISBN 0-916894-28-X
                    00028
0
  29129004495
```

UC Recopy: _____

Date / Exp.	MEDICATION ADMINISTRATION RECORD SCHEDULED: A	24 01 02 03	04 05 06 07	08 09 10 11	12 13 14 15	16 17 18 19	20 21 22 23	RN ✓	Date 6/10/XX			Date 6/11			Date 6/12		
									23	07	15	23	07	15	23	07	15
6/10	~~hydralazine 25 mg PO q6~~ *mistaken entry Juni R. 11/15/18*																
	~~until itching subsides~~																
	hydroxyzine 25mg PO prn for itching																

Steps for Correcting a Written Error on a Chart Form

1. Draw one single line in ink through the error. ❏

⭐ **HIGH PRIORITY**

When only a single line is used to cancel the error, the original information is still readable. When correcting an error on the MAR, the line is drawn through the order date and the name of the medication through the end of the documentation dates.

2. Write the words "mistaken entry" in ink above or next to the error. ❏

3. Write the date, time, your first initial, your last name, and your status in a blank area near the words "mistaken entry." ❏

4. Write the correct order on line 2. ❏

Place a check mark (✓) in the following box to indicate that you have completed Activity 8-7.

❏ Correct a Written Error on a Chart Form   Date: _____

CHAPTER 10

Patient Activity, Patient Positioning, and Nursing Observation Orders

Activities in this Chapter:

10–1: Transcribe a Patient Activity Order

10–2: Transcribe a Patient Positioning Order

10–3: Transcribe Nursing Observation Orders

10–4: Transcribe a Blood Glucose Monitoring Order

10–5: Automatically Cancel and Discontinue Doctors' Orders

10–6: Transcribe a Review Set of Doctors' Orders

10–7: Transcribe Recorded Telephone Messages

★ HIGH PRIORITY

When an electronic medical record (EMR) with computerized physician order entry system has been implemented, doctors will enter orders directly into patients' EMRs. The responsibilities of the HUC will change from transcribing handwritten doctors' orders to monitoring the EMRs for HUC tasks (indicated by an icon). The activities in this and subsequent chapters provide an understanding of patient care and will prepare you to work in health care facilities that use the paper chart or the EMR system.

★ HIGH PRIORITY

Review Chapter 10 in *LaFleur Brooks' Health Unit Coordinating*, 7th edition, for explanations of doctors' orders and definitions of abbreviations.

Place the Physicians' Order Sheets located at the end of the chapter in your patient's chart. Follow the directions for each activity to transcribe orders.

ACTIVITY 10-1

TRANSCRIBE A PATIENT ACTIVITY ORDER

Materials Needed

Black ink pen

Red ink pen (depending on hospital policy)

Pencil

Eraser

Kardex form

Physicians' order sheets located at the end of this chapter (placed in your patient's chart)

Computer with Practice Activity Software for Transcription of Physicians' Orders

Directions

Refer to Physicians' Order Sheet 10-1 in your patient's chart. Label or write your patient's name at the top of the order sheet. Write the date and time in the left column next to the first order and sign the name of the patient's doctor after "Dr" at the bottom of the order sheet. Practice transcribing the patient activity order by following the steps below. Check with your instructor for variations of the procedure to adapt the procedure to the practice in your area. Place a check mark (✓) in the box as you complete each step.

★ HIGH PRIORITY

Recite all 5 steps of transcription to yourself as you transcribe the orders to ensure that you do not miss a step. Not every set of orders requires all 5 steps.

Steps for Transcribing a Patient Activity Order

1. Read the order. ☐

2. Obtain the Kardex form. ☐

3. Document the order by:
   a. writing the date and the activity order in pencil in the activity column on the Kardex form ☐
   b. writing "K" in ink in the symbol column in front of the order on the doctor's order sheet to indicate completion of the documentation ☐

★ HIGH PRIORITY

The Kardex form used in this activity will be used through Chapter 18 as a Kardex form would be used during a patient's admission. You will be erasing, changing, and adding information as the doctor's orders are transcribed. It is important to write small, neatly, and legibly and to have a no. 2 pencil with a good eraser or a separate eraser.

4. Recheck each step for accuracy. ☐

5. Sign off the order in ink by writing the following on the line directly below the doctor's signature (begin on the left margin):
   a. the date ☐
   b. the time ☐
   c. your full signature ☐
   d. your status ☐

> ### ★ HIGH PRIORITY
>
> Color of ink used to document completion of transcription steps may be black or red (depends on hospital policy). Blue is not used because it does not copy well.

> ### ★ HIGH PRIORITY
>
> Signing off on a set of orders on the line directly below the doctor's signature avoids leaving space that could be used by the doctor to write additional orders at a later date that could be overlooked.

Place a check mark (✓) in the following box to indicate that you have completed Activity 10-1.

☐ Transcribe a Patient Activity Order   Date: _____

◎ ACTIVITY 10-2

TRANSCRIBE A PATIENT POSITIONING ORDER

Materials Needed   Black ink pen

Red ink pen (depending on hospital policy)

Pencil

Eraser

Kardex form used for Activity 10-1

Directions

Refer to Physicians' Order Sheet 10-2 in your patient's chart. Label or write your patient's name at the top of the order sheet. Write the date and time in the left column next to the first order and sign the name of the patient's doctor after "Dr" at the bottom of the order sheet. Practice transcribing the patient positioning order by performing the following steps. Check with your instructor for variations of the procedure to adapt the procedure to the practice in your area. Place a check mark (✓) in the box as you complete each step.

Steps for Transcribing a Patient Positioning Order

1. Read the order.   ☐

2. Obtain the Kardex form.   ☐

3. Document the order by:
   a. writing the date and the positioning order in pencil in the activity column on the Kardex form   ☐
   b. writing "K" in ink in the symbol column in front of the order on the doctor's order sheet to indicate completion of the documentation   ☐

4. Recheck each step for accuracy.   ☐

5. Sign off the order in ink by writing the following on the line directly below the doctor's signature (begin on the left margin):
   a. the date   ☐
   b. the time   ☐
   c. your full signature   ☐
   d. your status   ☐

Place a check mark (✓) in the following box to indicate that you have completed Activity 10-2.

❏ Transcribe a Patient Positioning Order   Date: _____

ACTIVITY 10-3

TRANSCRIBE NURSING OBSERVATION ORDERS

Materials Needed   Black ink pen
Red ink pen (depending on hospital policy)
Pencil
Eraser
Kardex form used in Activities 10-1 and 10-2

Directions

Refer to Physicians' Order Sheet 10-3 in your patient's chart. Label or write your patient's name at the top of the order sheet. Write the date and time in the left column next to the first order and sign the name of the patient's doctor after "Dr" at the bottom of the order sheet. Practice transcribing the nursing observation orders by performing the following steps. Check with your instructor for variations of the procedure to adapt the procedure to the practice in your area. Place a check mark (✓) in the box as you complete each step.

Steps for Transcribing Nursing Observation Orders

1. Read the orders.   ❏

2. Obtain the Kardex form.   ❏

3. Document the orders by:
   a. writing the date and orders in pencil in the appropriate column on the Kardex form (usually
      the column has the same heading as the doctor's order sheet)   ❏
   b. writing the symbol "K" in ink in front of the orders on the doctor's order sheet to indicate
      completion of the documentation   ❏

4. Recheck each step for accuracy.   ❏

5. Sign off the orders in ink by writing the following on the line directly below the doctor's signature
      (begin on the left margin):
   a. the date   ❏
   b. the time   ❏
   c. your full signature   ❏
   d. your status   ❏

Place a check mark (✓) in the following box to indicate that you have completed Activity 10-3.

❏ Transcribe Nursing Observation Orders   Date: _____

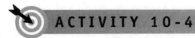

ACTIVITY 10-4

TRANSCRIBE A BLOOD GLUCOSE MONITORING ORDER

Materials Needed   Black ink pen

Red ink pen (depending on hospital policy)

Pencil

Eraser

Kardex form used in Activities 10-1 through 10-3

Directions

Refer to Physicians' Order Sheet 10-4 in your patient's chart. Label or write your patient's name at the top of the order sheet. Write the date and time in the left column next to the first order and sign the name of the patient's doctor after "Dr" at the bottom of the order sheet. Practice transcribing the blood glucose monitoring order by performing the following steps. Check with your instructor for variations of the procedure to adapt the procedure to the practice in your area. Place a check mark (✓) in the box as you complete each step.

Steps for Transcribing a Blood Glucose Monitoring Order

1. Read the order.   ☐

2. Obtain the Kardex form.   ☐

3. Document the order by:
   a. writing the date and the order in pencil in the treatment column on the Kardex form   ☐
   b. writing "K" in ink in the symbol column in front of the order on the doctor's order sheet to indicate completion of the documentation   ☐

4. Recheck each step for accuracy.   ☐

5. Sign off the orders in ink by writing the following on the line directly below the doctor's signature (begin on the left margin):
   a. the date   ☐
   b. the time   ☐
   c. your full signature   ☐
   d. your status   ☐

Place a check mark (✓) in the following box to indicate that you have completed Activity 10-4.

☐ Transcribe a Blood Glucose Monitoring Order   Date: _____

ACTIVITY 10-5

AUTOMATICALLY CANCEL AND DISCONTINUE DOCTORS' ORDERS

Materials Needed   Black ink pen

Red ink pen (depending on hospital policy)

Pencil

Eraser

Kardex form used in Activities 10-1 through 10-4

Directions

Refer to Physicians' Order Sheet 10-5 in your patient's chart. Label or write your patient's name at the top of the order sheet. Write the date and time in the left column next to the first order and sign the name of the patient's doctor after "Dr" at the bottom of the order sheet. Practice transcribing the orders by performing the following steps. Check with your instructor for variations of the procedure to adapt the procedure to the practice in your area. Place a check mark (✓) in the box as you complete each step.

Steps for Automatically Canceling and Discontinuing Doctors' Orders

1. Read the orders.   ☐

2. Obtain the Kardex form.   ☐

3. Document the discontinued orders by:
  a. erasing the existing date and order   ☐
  b. writing "K" in ink in the symbol column in front of the order on the doctor's order sheet to indicate completion of the documentation   ☐

4. Document the automatically cancelled orders by:
  a. erasing the existing date and order   ☐
  b. writing the date and new order in pencil in the appropriate column on the Kardex form   ☐
  c. writing "K" in ink in the symbol column in front of the order on the doctor's order sheet to indicate completion of the documentation   ☐

> ★ **HIGH PRIORITY**
>
> When a doctor changes an existing order, the new order will automatically cancel the existing order.

5. Recheck each step for accuracy.   ☐

6. Sign off the orders in ink by writing the following on the line directly below the doctor's signature (begin at the left margin):
  a. the date   ☐
  b. the time   ☐
  c. your full signature   ☐
  d. your status   ☐

Place a check mark (✓) in the following box to indicate that you have completed Activity 10-5.

☐ Automatically Cancel and Discontinue Doctors' Orders   Date: _____

◎ ACTIVITY 10-6

TRANSCRIBE A REVIEW SET OF DOCTORS' ORDERS

Materials Needed   Black ink pen

Red ink pen (depending on hospital policy)

Pencil

Eraser

Kardex form used in Activity 10-1 through 10-5

Directions

Refer to Physicians' Order Sheet 10-6 in your patient's chart. Transcribe the orders. Refer to previous activities for the appropriate directions to prepare for the transcription.

Steps for Transcribing a Review Set of Doctors' Orders

1. Read the orders. ❏

2. Obtain all necessary forms. ❏

Suggestion to the student: Use this space to list the forms you will need.

---

3. Document the orders on the Kardex form. ❏

4. Recheck each step for accuracy. ❏

5. Sign off the orders to indicate completion of transcription. ❏

⭐ **HIGH PRIORITY**

Transcribing doctors' orders is a critical task. An error could cause harm to a patient. If not absolutely sure when interpreting a doctor's order, ask the patient's nurse or the doctor who wrote the orders.

Place a check mark (✓) in the following box to indicate that you have completed Activity 10-6.

❏ Transcribe a Review Set of Doctors' Orders   Date: _____

⦿ **ACTIVITY 10-7**

TRANSCRIBE RECORDED TELEPHONE MESSAGES

Note: Transcribing recorded telephone messages is an important part of the HUC's job. Activities for practice in transcribing recorded messages are provided in this chapter and in subsequent chapters through Chapter 18.

Materials Needed   Pen or pencil
                              Note pad

Directions

Practice transcribing the following telephone messages by following the steps listed. Place a check mark (✓) in the box as you complete each step.

Telephone Messages

1. "Hello, this is Dr. Peterson. Would you ask Mrs. Johnson's nurse (Diane) to call me for orders regarding medication changes? My back office number is 345-4980. Thank you."

2. "Hi, this is Jamie from Dr. Sanburn's office. Dr. Sanburn would like the nurse to call regarding Johnny Appleton. Our number is 596-3249."

Steps for Transcribing Telephone Messages

1. Have someone read these messages to you while you write them on a note pad. ❑

2. Write down for whom the message is intended. ❑

3. Write down the caller's name. ❑

4. Write down the date and time of the call. ❑

5. Write down the purpose of the call. ❑

6. If a return call is expected, write down the number to call. ❑

7. Sign your name to the message. ❑

Place a check mark (✓) in the following box to indicate that you have completed Activity 10-7.

❑ Transcribe Recorded Telephone Messages   Date: _____

CHAPTER 11

Nursing Treatment Orders

Activities in this Chapter:

★ HIGH PRIORITY

When an electronic medical record (EMR) with computerized physician order entry system has been implemented, doctors will enter orders directly into patients' EMRs. The responsibilities of the health unit coordinator (HUC) will change from transcribing the handwritten doctors' orders to monitoring the EMRs for HUC tasks (indicated by an icon, usually a telephone). The nurse may also request that the HUC order supplies or equipment or place calls. The activities in this and subsequent chapters provide an understanding of patient care and prepare you to work in health care facilities that use the paper chart or the EMR system.

★ HIGH PRIORITY

Paper requisitions are seldom used, even when paper charts are used, because computer maintenance downtime is usually scheduled at night when few orders are written. The procedure for using paper requisitions is included in this chapter to assist you in learning the supplies and equipment needed for various treatments and procedures and how to order them. The Practice Activity Software for Transcription of Physicians' Orders provides practice ordering supplies and equipment via computer.

The purpose of the ordering step is to forward the doctors' orders to the hospital departments that will execute the orders.

> ⭐ **HIGH PRIORITY**
>
> Review Chapter 11 in *LaFleur Brooks' Health Unit Coordinating*, 7th edition, for explanations of doctors' orders and definitions of abbreviations.

> Place the Physicians' Order Sheets located at the end of the chapter in your patient's chart. Follow the directions for each activity to transcribe orders.

 ACTIVITY 11-1

TRANSCRIBE URINARY CATHETERIZATION AND INTESTINAL ELIMINATION ORDERS

Materials Needed

Black ink pen

Red ink pen (depending on hospital policy)

Pencil

Eraser

Kardex form used in Chapter 10

Physicians' order sheets located at the end of this chapter (placed in your patient's chart)

Directions

Refer to Physicians' Order Sheet 11-1 in your patient's chart. Practice transcribing the nursing treatment orders by performing the following steps. Check with your instructor for variations of the procedure to adapt it to the practice in your area. Place a check mark (✓) in the box as you complete each step.

Steps for Transcribing Urinary Catheterization and Intestinal Elimination Orders

1. Read the orders. ☐

2. Obtain the Kardex form used in Chapter 10. ☐

3. Document the orders by:
   a. writing the date and order in pencil in the treatment column on the Kardex form ☐
   b. writing "K" in ink in the symbol column in front of the order on the doctor's order sheet to indicate completion of the documentation ☐

4. Recheck each step for accuracy. ☐

5. Sign off the orders to indicate completion of transcription. ☐

Place a check mark (✔) in the following box to indicate that you have completed Activity 11-1.

☐ Transcribe Urinary Catheterization and Intestinal Elimination Orders

Date: _____

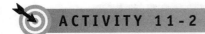

ACTIVITY 11-2

TRANSCRIBE INTRAVENOUS THERAPY ORDERS

Materials Needed   Black ink pen

Red ink pen (depending on hospital policy)

Pencil

Eraser

Kardex form used in Activity 11-1

Patient ID labels (if using requisitions)

Central service department (CSD) requisition form (if using requisitions) or computer and Practice Activity Software for Transcription of Physicians' Orders on Evolve

Directions

Refer to Physicians' Order Sheet 11-2 in your patient's chart. Practice transcribing the nursing treatment orders by performing the following steps. Check with your instructor for variations of the procedure to adapt it to the practice in your area. Place a check mark (✓) in the box as you complete each step.

Steps for Transcribing Intravenous Therapy Orders

1. Read the orders. ☐

2. Obtain the Kardex form and a CSD requisition form if using the requisition method. ☐

3. Order an intravenous (IV) infusion pump. ☐

★ HIGH PRIORITY

When using a hospital computer to complete the ordering step, press enter after completing the order screen to send the order to the appropriate department. An order number will appear on the screen when the order has been entered; write this number above each item ordered (this is in place of writing "ord").

---

4. Use the computer and the practice software by:
   a. selecting Enter Orders on the home screen ☐
   b. selecting the patient's name from the census on the viewing screen ☐
   c. selecting Central Service from the department menu on the viewing screen ☐
   d. selecting the IV infusion pump from the menu on the viewing screen ☐
   e. typing in the pertinent information ☐

5. Use the requisition form by:
   a. affixing the patient's label to the form ☐
   b. filling in the pertinent information ☐
   c. writing the number "1" in the box next to "IV infusion pump" (in ink) ☐
   d. writing "ord IV pump" above the IV order on the doctor's order sheet to indicate that the IV equipment has been ordered ☐

6. Document the orders by:
   a. writing the date and the order in pencil in the IV column on the Kardex form ☐
   b. writing "K" in ink in the symbol column in front of the order on the doctor's order sheet to indicate completion of the documentation ☐

7. Recheck each step for accuracy. ☐

8. Sign off the orders to indicate completion of transcription. ☐

> ## ★ HIGH PRIORITY
>
> Some hospitals may use a parenteral fluid or infusion form to record IV orders, and some may write the IV orders on the medication administration record.

Place a check mark (✔) in the following box to indicate that you have completed Activity 11-2.

❏ Transcribe IV Therapy Orders   Date: _____

◎ ACTIVITY 11-3

TRANSCRIBE SUCTION ORDERS

Materials Needed   Black ink pen

Red ink pen (depending on hospital policy)

Pencil

Eraser

Kardex form used in Activity 11-2

List of items that may be stored in the CSD (see Table 11-1 in *LaFleur Brooks' Health Unit Coordinating,* 7th edition)

Patient ID label (if using requisitions)

CSD requisition form (if using requisitions) or computer and Practice Activity Software for Transcription of Physicians' Orders

Directions

Refer to Physicians' Order Sheet 11-3 in your patient's chart. Practice transcribing the nursing treatment orders by performing the following steps. Check with your instructor for variations of the procedure to adapt it to the practice in your area. Place a check mark (✓) in the box as you complete each step.

Steps for Transcribing Suction Orders

1. Read the orders.   ❏

2. Obtain the Kardex form and a CSD requisition form if using the requisition method.   ❏

> ## ★ HIGH PRIORITY
>
> Refer to Table 11-1 in *LaFleur Brooks' Health Unit Coordinating,* 7th edition, to determine the supplies and equipment that may need to be ordered.

3. Order the supplies and equipment from the CSD.   ❏

Use the computer and the practice software by:

    a. selecting Enter Orders from the home screen   ❏

    b. selecting the patient's name from the census on the viewing screen   ❏

    c. selecting Central Service from the department menu on the viewing screen   ❏

    d. selecting the items to be ordered from the menu on the viewing screen and typing in the pertinent information   ❏

    e. sending the order by pressing Enter Order(s) on the viewing screen   ❏

Use the requisition form by:
   a. affixing the patient's label to the form   ❑
   b. filling in the pertinent information   ❑
   c. writing an "X" or a quantity (if applicable) in the column next to the items to be ordered   ❑
   d. writing "ord" in ink above any item ordered on the doctor's order sheet to indicate that the item was ordered   ❑

★ HIGH PRIORITY

Writing the order number as it appears on the computer screen or "ord" above each item ordered will reduce the risk of missing items.
    Example: ord
    K-pad to lower lt arm 20 min qid

---

4. Document the orders by:
   a. writing the date and order in pencil in the treatment column on the Kardex form   ❑
   b. writing "K" in ink in the symbol column in front of the order on the doctor's order sheet to indicate completion of the documentation   ❑
5. Recheck each step for accuracy.   ❑
6. Sign off the orders to indicate completion of transcription.   ❑

Place a check mark (✓) in the following box to indicate that you have completed Activity 11-3.

❑ Transcribe Suction Orders   Date: _____

◎ ACTIVITY 11-4

TRANSCRIBE HEAT AND COLD APPLICATION ORDERS AND COMFORT, SAFETY, AND HEALING ORDERS

Materials Needed   Black ink pen
                       Red ink pen (depending on hospital policy)
                       Pencil
                       Eraser
                       Kardex form used in Activity 11-3
                       Patient ID labels (when using the requisition method)
                       CSD requisition form (if using requisitions) or computer and Practice Activity Software for Transcription of Physicians' Orders

Directions

Refer to Physicians' Order Sheet 11-4 in your patient's chart. Practice transcribing the nursing treatment orders by performing the following steps. Check with your instructor for variations of the procedure to adapt it to the practice in your area. Place a check mark (✓) in the box as you complete each step.

Steps for Transcribing Heat and Cold Application Orders and Comfort, Safety, and Healing Orders

1. Read the orders.   ❑
2. Obtain the Kardex form and a CSD requisition form if using the requisition method.   ❑

> ⭐ **HIGH PRIORITY**
>
> Refer to Table 11-1 in *LaFleur Brooks' Health Unit Coordinating,* 7th edition, to determine the supplies and equipment that may need to be ordered.

---

3. Order the supplies and equipment from the CSD.   ❏

Use the computer and the practice software by:
   a. selecting Enter Orders from the home screen   ❏
   b. selecting the patient's name from the census on the viewing screen   ❏
   c. selecting Central Service from the department menu on the viewing screen   ❏
   d. selecting the items to be ordered from the menu on the viewing screen   ❏
   e. typing in the pertinent information   ❏
   f. sending the order by pressing Enter Order(s) on the viewing screen   ❏

Use the requisition form by:
   a. affixing the patient's label to the form   ❏
   b. filling in the pertinent information   ❏
   c. writing an "X" or a quantity (if applicable) in the column next to the items to be ordered   ❏
   d. writing "ord" in ink above each order on the doctor's order sheet to indicate that supplies and equipment have been ordered   ❏

4. Document the orders by:
   a. writing the date and order in pencil in the treatment column on the Kardex form   ❏
   b. writing "K" in ink in the symbol column in front of the order on the doctor's order sheet to indicate completion of the documentation   ❏

5. Recheck each step for accuracy.   ❏

6. Sign off the orders to indicate completion of transcription.   ❏

Place a check mark (✔) in the following box to indicate that you have completed Activity 11-4.

❏ Transcribe Heat and Cold Application Orders and
   Comfort, Safety, and Healing Orders   Date: _____

🎯 **ACTIVITY 11-5**

TRANSCRIBE A REVIEW SET OF DOCTORS' ORDERS

Materials Needed   Black ink pen

Red ink pen (depending on hospital policy)

Pencil

Eraser

Kardex form used in Activity 11-4

Patient ID label (if using requisitions)

Necessary requisition forms (if using requisitions) or computer and Practice Activity Software for Transcription of Physicians' Orders

Directions

Refer to Physicians' Order Sheet 11-5 in your patient's chart. Transcribe the orders. Review the previous activities for the appropriate transcription steps if necessary.

Steps for Transcribing a Review Set of Doctors' Orders

1. Read the orders.   ☐

2. Obtain all necessary forms.   ☐

Suggestion to the student: Use this space to list the forms you will need.

3. Order as necessary.   ☐

4. Document the orders on the Kardex form.   ☐

5. Recheck each step for accuracy.   ☐

6. Sign off the orders to indicate the completion of transcription.   ☐

(★) HIGH PRIORITY

Transcribing doctors' orders is a critical task. An error could cause harm to a patient. If you are not absolutely sure when interpreting the doctor's orders, ask the patient's nurse or the doctor who wrote the orders.

Place a check mark (✔) in the following box to indicate that you have completed Activity 11-5.

☐ Transcribe a Review Set of Doctors' Orders   Date: _____

(★) HIGH PRIORITY

Refer to Chapter 11 in *LaFleur Brooks' Health Unit Coordinating,* 7th edition, to determine how long the two bags of IV solution ordered in Activity 11-6 would take to infuse.

(◎) ACTIVITY 11-6

TRANSCRIBE RECORDED TELEPHONE MESSAGES

Materials Needed   Pen or pencil
Note pad

Directions

Practice transcribing the following recorded telephone messages by performing the steps that follow. Place a check mark (✔) in the box as you complete each step.

Telephone Messages

1. "Hello, this is Don in the CSD. Would you ask Mary Copa's nurse for a size on those TED hose that were ordered? All the requisition indicated was that they were to be thigh high, and we need to know a size." ❏

2. "This is Melba in the pharmacy. Please notify the resident for Peter Franks that we need a clarification on the chemotherapy orders before noon today. Fax them to us as soon as you have them. Thanks." ❏

Steps for Transcribing Telephone Messages

1. Have someone read these messages to you while you transcribe them on a note pad. ❏

2. Write down for whom the message is intended. ❏

3. Write down the caller's name. ❏

4. Write down the date and time of the call. ❏

5. Write down the purpose of the call. ❏

6. If a return call is expected, write down the number to call. ❏

7. Sign your name to the message. ❏

Place a check mark (✔) in the following box to indicate that you have completed Activity 11-6.

❏ Transcribe Recorded Telephone Messages   Date: _____

PHYSICIANS' ORDER SHEET 11-1

DATE	TIME	SYMBOL	ORDERS
			Fleets enema this am
			√ for residual
			Insert indwelling cath if residual > 100cc
			DC CMS fingers lt hand
			Dr.

PHYSICIANS' ORDER SHEET 11-2

DATE	TIME	SYMBOL	ORDERS
			Foley cath to con't drainage
			DC orthostatics
			Start IV stat
			Alt 1000cc D5LR c̄ 1000cc 0.45 NS @ 120cc/hr
			Call hospitalist if IV infiltrates
			Dr.

PHYSICIANS' ORDER SHEET 11-3

DATE	TIME	SYMBOL	ORDERS
			CBR
			VS q 4 hr until stable
			DC daily wt
			Insert chest tube with Pleur-evac @ 20cm H_2O
			suction rt side
			Δ IV to 1000 cc bag of NS @ 100 cc/hr
			Throat sx @ BS
			Dr.

PHYSICIANS' ORDER SHEET 11-4

DATE	TIME	SYMBOL	ORDERS
			Aquathermia pad @ med heat to lower back 20 min qid
			Ice bag to rt ankle as tol
			Sheepskin & footboard to bed
			Ted hose c̄ Pneumatic compression to lt calf
			TCDB q4° between 7 am and 11 pm
			Jacket restraint for agitation per protocol—have restraint
			form available
			Convert IV to HL c̄ rout saline flushes
			Dr.

PHYSICIANS' ORDER SHEET 11-5

DATE	TIME	SYMBOL	ORDERS
			DC jacket restraint
			Notify hospitalist if pt becomes agitated again
			May sit in chair 20 min bid
			Closely monitor pt when in chair
			Con't pneumatic compression to lt calf when in bed
			DC HL
			Insert PICC & start IVF of 0.45 NS @ 125cc/hr
			May shampoo hair
			VS q shift
			Dr.
			Remove indwelling cath in am. If unable to void in 6°, reinsert
			Dr.

CHAPTER **12**

Nutritional Care Orders

Activities in this Chapter:

12–1: Transcribe a Standard Hospital Diet Order
12–2: Transcribe a Therapeutic Diet Order
12–3: Transcribe a Tube-Feeding Order
12–4: Transcribe a Review Set of Doctors' Orders
12–5: Transcribe Recorded Telephone Messages

⭐ HIGH PRIORITY

When an electronic medical record (EMR) with computerized physician order entry system has been implemented, doctors enter orders directly into patients' EMRs. The orders are automatically sent to the nutritional care department. The health unit coordinator (HUC) may have the responsibility of ordering food trays for patients returning from procedures or completing tests that required them to fast. The HUC may also order food and beverages for unit supply.

⭐ HIGH PRIORITY

The procedure for using paper requisitions is included in this chapter to assist you in learning the various nutritional care orders and the equipment and supplies needed for tube feeding. The computer and Practice Activity Software for Transcription of Physicians' Orders will provide practice ordering diets, equipment, and supplies via computer.

⭐ HIGH PRIORITY

Review Chapter 12 in *LaFleur Brooks' Health Unit Coordinating*, 7th edition, for explanations of doctors' orders and definitions of abbreviations.

Place the Physicians' Order Sheets located at the end of this chapter in your patient's chart. Follow the directions for each activity to transcribe orders.

 ACTIVITY 12-1

TRANSCRIBE A STANDARD HOSPITAL DIET ORDER

Materials Needed
Black ink pen
Red ink pen (depending on hospital policy)
Pencil
Eraser
Kardex form used in previous chapters
Patient ID labels (if requisitions used)
Nutritional care requisition form (if requisitions used) or computer and Practice Activity Software for Transcription of Physicians' Orders

Directions

Refer to Physicians' Order Sheet 12-1 in your patient's chart. Practice transcribing the standard hospital diet by performing the following steps. Check with your instructor for variations of the procedure to adapt it to the practice in your area. Place a check mark (✓) in the box as you complete each step.

Steps for Transcribing a Standard Hospital Diet Order

1. Read the order. ☐

2. Obtain the Kardex form used in Chapter 11 and a dietary requisition form if using the requisition method. ☐

3. Order the diet from the nutritional care department. ☐

Use the computer and the practice software by:
a. selecting Enter Orders on the home screen ☐
b. selecting the patient's name from the census on the viewing screen ☐
c. selecting the nutritional care department from the department menu on the viewing screen ☐
d. selecting the diet to be ordered from the menu on the viewing screen ☐
e. typing in the pertinent information ☐
f. sending the order by pressing Enter Order(s) on the viewing screen ☐
g. writing "ord" in ink above the order on the doctor's order sheet to indicate that the diet has been ordered ☐

Use the requisition form by:
a. affixing the patient's ID label to the form ☐
b. writing in the pertinent information ☐
c. placing a check mark (✓) in the column next to the diet to be ordered ☐
d. writing "ord" in ink above the order on the doctor's order sheet to indicate that the diet has been ordered ☐

4. Document the order by:
a. writing the date and the order in pencil in the diet column on the Kardex form ☐
b. writing "K" in ink in the symbol column in front of the order on the doctor's order sheet to indicate completion of the documentation ☐

5. Recheck each step for accuracy. ☐

6. Sign off the order to indicate completion of transcription. ☐

Place a check mark (✓) in the following box to indicate that you have completed Activity 12-1.

☐ Transcribe a Standard Hospital Diet Order   Date: _____

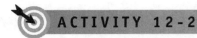

TRANSCRIBE A THERAPEUTIC DIET ORDER

Materials Needed   Black ink pen

Red ink pen (depending on hospital policy)

Pencil

Eraser

Kardex form used in Activity 12-1

Patient ID labels (if requisitions used)

Nutritional care requisition form (if requisitions used) or computer and Practice Activity Software for Transcription of Physicians' Orders

Directions

Refer to Physicians' Order Sheet 12-2 in your patient's chart. Practice transcribing the therapeutic diet order by performing the following steps. Check with your instructor for variations of the procedure to adapt it to the practice in your area. Place a check mark (✓) in the box as you complete each step.

> ★ **HIGH PRIORITY**
>
> An order modifying a nutrient or number of calories would *not* change the consistency of a patient's diet.
>   *Example:* If the patient is on a "soft diet" and the doctor wrote an order for "2 g Na," the patient's diet would then be a "soft 2 g Na."

Steps for Transcribing a Therapeutic Diet Order

1. Read the order. ☐

2. Obtain the Kardex form and a dietary requisition form if using the requisition method. ☐

3. Order the diet from the nutritional care department. ☐

Use the computer and the practice software by:
a. selecting Enter Orders on the home screen ☐
b. selecting the patient's name from the census on the viewing screen ☐
c. selecting the nutritional care department from the department menu on the viewing screen ☐
d. selecting the diet to be ordered from the menu on the viewing screen ☐
e. typing in the pertinent information ☐
f. sending the order by pressing Enter Order(s) on the viewing screen ☐
g. writing "ord" in ink above the order on the doctor's order sheet to indicate that the diet has been ordered ☐

Use the requisition form by:
a. affixing the patient's ID label to the form ☐
b. writing in the pertinent information ☐
c. placing a check mark (✓) in the column next to the diet to be ordered ☐
d. writing "ord" in ink above the order on the doctor's order sheet to indicate the diet has been ordered ☐

4. Document the order by:
a. writing the date and the order in pencil in the diet column on the Kardex form ☐
b. writing "K" in ink in the symbol column in front of the order on the doctor's order sheet to indicate completion of the documentation ☐

5. Recheck each step for accuracy. ☐

6. Sign off the order to indicate completion of transcription. ☐

Place a check mark (✓) in the following box to indicate that you have completed Activity 12-2.

☐ Transcribe a Therapeutic Diet Order   Date: _____

ACTIVITY 12-3

TRANSCRIBE A TUBE-FEEDING ORDER

Materials Needed   Black ink pen

Red ink pen (depending on hospital policy)

Pencil

Eraser

Kardex form used in Activity 12-2

Patient ID labels (if using requisitions)

Necessary requisition forms (if using requisitions) or computer and Practice Activity Software for Transcription of Physicians' Orders

Directions

Refer to Physicians' Order Sheet 12-3 in your patient's chart. Practice transcribing the tube-feeding order by performing the following steps. Check with your instructor for variations of the procedure to adapt it to the practice in your area. Place a check mark (✓) in the box as you complete each step.

> ### ★ HIGH PRIORITY
>
> The nurse may verify the tube placement by withdrawing a small amount of stomach contents or by using a syringe to inject air through the tube and listening with a stethoscope as the air enters the stomach.

Steps for Transcribing a Feeding-Tube Order

1. Read the order. ☐

2. Obtain the Kardex form and dietary requisition form if using the requisition method. ☐

3. Order the feeding pump with bag and tubing from the central service department (CSD). ☐

4. Order the tube-feeding formula from the nutritional care department. ☐

Use the computer and the practice software by:

a. selecting Enter Orders from the master screen ☐

b. selecting the patient's name from the census on the viewing screen ☐

c. selecting Central Service from the department menu on the viewing screen ☐

d. selecting the feeding pump with bag and tubing to be ordered ☐

e. typing in the pertinent information ☐

f. sending the order by pressing Enter Order(s) on the viewing screen ☐

g. writing "ord" in ink above the order on the doctor's order sheet to indicate that the feeding pump has been ordered ☐

h. selecting the nutritional care department from the department menu on the viewing screen ☐

i. selecting the Other option from the menu on the viewing screen and typing directions for the tube-feeding formula ☐

j. sending the order by pressing Enter Order(s) on the viewing screen ☐

k. writing "ord" in ink above the order on the doctor's order sheet to indicate that the tube-feeding formula has been ordered ☐

Use the requisition forms by:
a. affixing the patient's ID labels to the forms
b. writing in the pertinent information on the CSD requisition form
c. writing "ord" in ink above the order on the doctor's order sheet to indicate that the feeding pump and tubing have been ordered
d. writing in the pertinent information on the dietary requisition form
e. writing "ord" in ink above the order on the doctor's order sheet to indicate that the tube-feeding formula has been ordered

5. Document the order by:
a. writing the date and the order in pencil in the tube-feeding column on the Kardex form
b. writing "K" in ink in the symbol column in front of the order on the doctor's order sheet to indicate completion of the documentation

6. Recheck each step for accuracy.

7. Sign off on the order to indicate completion of transcription.

Place a check mark (✓) in the following box to indicate that you have completed Activity 12-3.

❑ Transcribe a Tube-Feeding Order   Date: _____

ACTIVITY 12-4

TRANSCRIBE A REVIEW SET OF DOCTORS' ORDERS

Materials Needed   Black ink pen

Red ink pen (depending on hospital policy)

Pencil

Eraser

Kardex form used in Activity 12-3

Necessary consent forms

Patient ID labels (if requisitions used)

Necessary requisition forms (if requisitions used) or computer and Practice Activity Software for Transcription of Physicians' Orders

Directions

Refer to Physicians' Order Sheet 12-4 in your patient's chart. Transcribe the orders. Refer to previous activities for the appropriate transcription steps if necessary.

Steps for Transcribing a Review Set of Doctors' Orders

1. Read the complete set of doctor's orders.

2. Obtain all necessary forms.

Suggestion to the student: Use this space to list the forms you will need.

3. Order as necessary.   ☐

4. Document the orders on the Kardex form.   ☐

5. Recheck each step for accuracy.   ☐

6. Sign off the orders to indicate completion of transcription.   ☐

★ HIGH PRIORITY

Transcribing doctors' orders is a critical task, and an error could cause harm to a patient. If you are not absolutely sure when interpreting the doctor's orders, ask the patient's nurse or the doctor who wrote the orders.

Place a check mark (✓) in the following box to indicate that you have completed Activity 12-4.

☐ Transcribe a Review Set of Doctors' Orders   Date: _____

◎ ACTIVITY 12-5

TRANSCRIBE RECORDED TELEPHONE MESSAGES

Materials Needed   Pen or pencil
Note pad

Directions

Practice transcribing the following telephone messages by performing the following steps. Place a check mark (✓) in the box as you complete each step.

Telephone Messages

1. "Hello, this is Charlotte Jones from APS. I'm arranging to have Paula Praline admitted to an adult crisis center. Would you have the case manager call me at 495-3947 as soon as possible? I need to know if Paula is still on tube feeding or if she has any other dietary restrictions. Thanks."   ☐

2. "Hello, this is Dr. Johnson. Would you please advise Pete Grime's nurse that I will be in to place a gastrostomy tube at 0830 tomorrow? Please tell her to have the consent signed and to have the tray with size 8 gloves at the bedside. Thank you."   ☐

Steps for Transcribing Recorded Telephone Messages

1. Have someone read these messages to you while you transcribe them onto a note pad.   ☐

2. Write down the person's name for whom the message is intended.   ☐

3. Write down the caller's name.   ☐

4. Write down the date and time of the call.   ☐

5. Write down the purpose of the call.   ☐

6. If a return call is expected, write down the number to call.   ☐

7. Sign your name to the message.   ☐

Place a check mark (✓) in the following box to indicate that you have completed Activity 12-5.

☐ Transcribe Recorded Telephone Messages   Date: _____

PHYSICIANS' ORDER SHEET 12-1

DATE	TIME	SYMBOL	ORDERS
01/22		K	Allergy to peanuts
		K	Soft 1500 cal ADA diet
			Dr.

PHYSICIANS' ORDER SHEET 12-2

DATE	TIME	SYMBOL	ORDERS
01/22			1 g Na diet
01/23			Cal ct
01/23			RD to consult
			Dr.

PHYSICIANS' ORDER SHEET 12-3

DATE	TIME	SYMBOL	ORDERS
01/24		K	D/C PO diet
		K, ORD	Insert NG tube, verify placement, & begin tube
		K	feeding of Boost Plus full strength @ 35cc/hr,
		K	progress by 10cc/hr q4h as tol to final rate of 75cc/hr
			Dr.

PHYSICIANS' ORDER SHEET 12-4

DATE	TIME	SYMBOL	ORDERS
			DC chest tube & throat sx
			DC feeding tube & start on cl liq & adv DAT—1200 cal ADA
			diet
			Limit total fluids to 2500cc per day
			Encourage amb c̄ help
			If pt c/o of N/V, call Dr. Peterson stat
			Dr.

CHAPTER 13

Medication Orders

Activities in this Chapter:

★ HIGH PRIORITY

When the electronic medical record (EMR) with computerized physician order entry (CPOE) system has been implemented, transcription of doctors' medication orders will not be the responsibility of the HUC. Medication orders will be sent automatically to the hospital pharmacy as doctors enter the orders. The medications will also be listed on the patients' medication administration records (MARs) in their EMRs. The HUC will monitor the patients' EMRs and will complete specific HUC tasks indicated by an icon, such as a telephone. The HUC may also be responsible for instructing or assisting the physician or nurse in the use of the computer system.

HIGH PRIORITY

When the EMR with CPOE system has been implemented, it is still important for the HUC to have a basic knowledge of medications. The HUC may be responsible for printing patients' discharge instructions, prescriptions, and information sheets for each medication when patients are discharged.

 HIGH PRIORITY

In some hospitals that have not implemented the EMR with CPOE system, the pharmacy will send a printed MAR each morning for each patient to the nursing unit. If any new medications are ordered during the day, they will be handwritten on that MAR by the patient's nurse or the HUC. The doctor's orders for newly ordered medications are faxed to the pharmacy and will be added to the printed MAR the following day.

 HIGH PRIORITY

Review Chapter 13 in *LaFleur Brooks' Health Unit Coordinating*, 7th edition, for explanations of medications and definitions of abbreviations.
   The following activities provide practice in transcribing medication orders as well as assist one in becoming familiar with the names and uses of medications.

Place the Physicians' Order Sheets located at the end of this chapter in your patient's chart. Follow the directions for each activity to transcribe orders.

 ACTIVITY 13-1

TRANSCRIBE STANDING MEDICATION ORDERS

Materials Needed   Black ink pen

Red ink pen (depending on hospital policy)

Physicians' Desk Reference or pharmacology reference material

Medication time schedule (Table 13-2 in *LaFleur Brooks' Health Unit Coordinating*, 7th edition)

Labeled MAR

Computer and Practice Activity Software for Transcription of Physicians' Orders

Directions

Refer to Physicians' Order Sheet 13-1 in your patient's chart. Practice transcribing the standing medication orders by performing the following steps. Check with your instructor for variations of this procedure to adapt it to the practice in your area. Place a check mark ✓ in the box as you complete each step.

 HIGH PRIORITY

The MAR used in this activity is used in all of the following activities. Medications that are not changed or discontinued are copied on a new MAR when all lines have been used.

Steps for Transcribing Standing Medication Orders

1. Read the orders.

> **★ HIGH PRIORITY**
>
> Use the *Physicians' Desk Reference* or other pharmacology reference material to become familiar with the purpose and the correct spelling of medications.

> **★ HIGH PRIORITY**
>
> Some medications are administered by one route only. Therefore the doctor may not include the route of administration when writing the order.

2. Obtain the MAR.

3. Order medications by faxing or sending the pharmacy copy of the doctor's orders to the pharmacy.

> **★ HIGH PRIORITY**
>
> Medications are ordered by faxing or sending a copy of the doctor's orders to the pharmacy. It may not be possible to practice this step in the classroom. Follow the next step of writing "faxed pc" (faxed pharmacy copy) or "pcs" (pharmacy copy sent) with the time and your initials to indicate that the task has been completed.

4. Write "faxed pc" or "pcs" with the time and your initials in ink on the doctor's order sheet to indicate that the pharmacy copy has been sent.

> **★ HIGH PRIORITY**
>
> It is important to send pharmacy copies or to fax doctors' orders to the pharmacy as soon as possible so medications can then be sent to the department and be administered to patients. If several charts are flagged, read all orders, transcribe "stat" orders, and send pharmacy copies or fax orders before beginning the transcription of orders (one chart at a time).

5. Enter medications on your patient's medication profile by using a computer and the practice software by:
   a. typing (1) today's date; (2) the name of the medication and dosage; (3) the route; (4) the frequency; (5) and the qualifying phrase, if used (refer to Table 13-2 in *LaFleur Brooks' Health Unit Coordinating,* 7th edition)

OR

Document the medications in ink on the MAR under the correct heading (standing, prn, state, etc.) by:
   a. writing (1) today's date; (2) the name of the medication and dosage; (3) the route; (4) the frequency; (5) and the qualifying phrase, if used (refer to Table 13-2 in *LaFleur Brooks' Health Unit Coordinating,* 7th edition)

> ★ **HIGH PRIORITY**
>
> Some health care facilities prefer that the nurse fill in the specific time of administration. The times may vary because of type of medication, patient's home schedule, or patient's eating schedule (particularly in pediatrics departments).

    b. writing "m" in ink in the symbol column in front of the order on the doctor's order sheet to indicate completion of the documentation ☐

6. Recheck each step for accuracy. ☐

7. Sign off the orders to indicate completion of transcription. ☐

Place a check mark (✓) in the following box to indicate that you have completed Activity 13-1.

☐ Transcribe Standing Medication Orders   Date: _____

◎ ACTIVITY 13-2

TRANSCRIBE PRN MEDICATION ORDERS

Materials Needed   Black ink pen

Red ink pen (depending on hospital policy)

Physicians' Desk Reference or pharmacology reference material

Medication time schedule (Table 13-2 in *LaFleur Brooks' Health Unit Coordinating,* 7th edition)

MAR used in Activity 13-1

Computer and Practice Activity Software for Transcription of Physicians' Orders

Directions

Refer to Physicians' Order Sheet 13-2 in your patient's chart. Practice transcribing the standing prn medication orders by performing the following steps. Check with your instructor for variations of this procedure to adapt it to the practice in your area. Place a check mark (✓) in the box as you complete each step.

Steps for Transcribing PRN Medication Orders

1. Read the orders. ☐

2. Obtain the MAR. ☐

3. Order medications by faxing or sending the pharmacy copy of the doctor's orders to the pharmacy. ☐

4. Write "faxed pc" or "pcs" with the time and your initials in ink on the doctor's order sheet to indicate that the pharmacy copy has been sent. ☐

5. Enter medications on your patient's medication profile by using a computer and the practice software by:

    a. typing in (1) today's date; (2) the name of the medication and dosage; (3) the route; (4) the frequency; (5) and the qualifying phrase, if used ☐

OR

Document the medications in ink on the MAR under the correct heading (standing, prn, stat, etc.) by:

    a. writing (1) today's date; (2) the name of the medication and dosage; (3) the route; (4) the frequency; (5) and the qualifying phrase, if used ☐

    b. writing "m" in ink in the symbol column in front of the order on the doctor's order sheet to indicate completion of the documentation ☐

6. Recheck each step for accuracy. ❑

7. Sign off the orders to indicate completion of transcription. ❑

Place a check mark (✓) in the following box to indicate that you have completed Activity 13-2.

❑ Transcribe PRN Medication Orders   Date: _____

⊚ ACTIVITY 13-3

TRANSCRIBE ONE-TIME MEDICATION ORDERS

Materials Needed   Black ink pen

Red ink pen (depending on hospital policy)

Physicians' Desk Reference or pharmacology reference material

Medication time schedule (Table 13-2 in *LaFleur Brooks' Health Unit Coordinating*, 7th edition)

MAR used in activity 13-2

Computer and Practice Activity Software for Transcription of Physicians' Orders

Directions

Refer to Physicians' Order Sheet 13-3 in your patient's chart. Practice transcribing the one-time medication orders by performing the following steps. Check with your instructor for variations of the procedure to adapt it to the practice in your area. Place a check mark (✓) in the box as you complete each step.

Steps for Transcribing One-Time Medication Orders

1. Read the orders. ❑

2. Obtain the MAR. ❑

3. Order medications by faxing or sending the pharmacy copy of the doctor's orders to the pharmacy. ❑

4. Write "faxed pc" or "pcs" with the time and your initials in ink on the doctor's order sheet to indicate that the pharmacy copy has been sent. ❑

5. Enter medications on your patient's medication profile by using a computer and the practice software by:
    a. typing in (1) today's date; (2) the name of the medication and dosage; (3) the route; (4) the frequency; (5) and the qualifying phrase, if used ❑

OR

Document the medications in ink on the MAR under the correct heading (standing, prn, stat, etc.) by:
    a. writing (1) today's date; (2) the name of the medication and dosage; (3) the route; (4) the frequency; (5) and the qualifying phrase, if used ❑
    b. writing "m" in ink in the symbol column in front of the order on the doctor's order sheet to indicate completion of the documentation ❑

6. Recheck each step for accuracy. ❑

7. Sign off the orders to indicate completion of transcription. ❑

Place a check mark (✓) in the following box to indicate that you have completed Activity 13-3.

❑ Transcribe One-Time Medication Orders   Date: _____

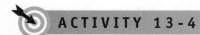
ACTIVITY 13-4

TRANSCRIBE SHORT-ORDER SERIES MEDICATION ORDERS

Materials Needed   Black ink pen

Red ink pen (depending on hospital policy)

Physicians' Desk Reference or pharmacology reference material

Medication time schedule (Table 13-2 in *LaFleur Brooks' Health Unit Coordinating,* 7th edition)

MAR used in activity 13-3

Computer and Practice Activity Software for Transcription of Physicians' Orders

Directions

Refer to Physicians' Order Sheet 13-4 on your patient's chart. Practice transcribing the short-order medication orders by performing the following steps. Check with your instructor for variations of the procedure to adapt it to the practice in your area. Place a check mark (✓) in the box as you complete each step.

Steps for Transcribing Short-Order Medication Orders

1. Read the orders. ☐

2. Obtain the MAR. ☐

3. Order medications by faxing or sending the pharmacy copy of the doctor's orders to the pharmacy. ☐

4. Write "faxed pc" or "pcs" with the time and your initials in ink on the doctor's order sheet to indicate that the pharmacy copy has been sent. ☐

5. Enter medications on your patient's medication profile by using a computer and the practice software by:
   a. typing in (1) today's date; (2) the name of the medication and dosage; (3) the route; (4) the frequency; (5) and the qualifying phrase, if used (refer to Table 13-2 in *LaFleur Brooks' Health Unit Coordinating,* 7th edition) ☐

OR

Document the medications in ink on the MAR under the correct heading (standing, prn, state, etc.) by:
   a. writing (1) today's date; (2) the name of the medication and dosage; (3) the route; (4) the frequency; (5) and the qualifying phrase, if used (refer to Table 13-2 in *LaFleur Brooks' Health Unit Coordinating,* 7th edition) ☐
   b. writing "m" in ink in the symbol column in front of the order on the doctor's order sheet to indicate completion of the documentation ☐

6. Recheck each step for accuracy. ☐

7. Sign off the orders to indicate completion of transcription. ☐

Place a check mark (✓) in the following box to indicate that you have completed Activity 13-4.

☐ Transcribe Short-Order Medication Orders   Date: _____

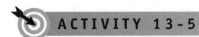

ACTIVITY 13-5

TRANSCRIBE STAT MEDICATION ORDERS

Materials Needed   Black ink pen

Red ink pen (depending on hospital policy)

Physicians' Desk Reference or pharmacology reference material

Medication time schedule (Table 13-2 in *LaFleur Brooks' Health Unit Coordinating*, 7th edition)

MAR used in activity 13-4

Computer and Practice Activity Software for Transcription of Physicians' Orders

Directions

Refer to Physicians' Order Sheet 13-5 in your patient's chart. Practice transcribing the stat medication orders by performing the following steps. Check with your instructor for variations of the procedure to adapt it to the practice in your area. Place a check mark (✓) in the box as you complete each step.

Steps for Transcribing Stat Medication Orders

1. Read the orders.   ❑

> ### ★ HIGH PRIORITY
>
> In the hospital setting, communicate a stat medication order at once by notifying the nurse responsible for administering the medication to the patient. Write "[name of nurse] notified" with the time and your initials on the order sheet.

2. Notify the appropriate nurse and write "nurse notified" with the time above the stat order.   ❑

3. Obtain the MAR.   ❑

4. Order medications by faxing or sending the pharmacy copy of the doctor's orders to the pharmacy.   ❑

5. Write "faxed pc" or "pcs" with the time and your initials in ink on the doctor's order sheet to indicate that the pharmacy copy has been sent.   ❑

6. Document the medications in ink on the MAR under the correct heading by:
   a. writing (1) today's date; (2) the name of the medication; (3) the dosage; (4) the route of administration   ❑

OR

Document the medications in ink on the MAR under the correct heading (standing, prn, state, etc.) by:
   a. writing (1) today's date; (2) the name of the medication; (3) the dosage; (4) the route of administration   ❑
   b. writing "m" in ink in the symbol column in front of the order on the doctor's order sheet to indicate completion of the documentation   ❑

7. Recheck each step for accuracy.   ❑

8. Sign off the orders to indicate completion of transcription.   ❑

Place a check mark (✓) in the following box to indicate that you have completed Activity 13-5.

❑ Transcribe Stat Medication Orders   Date: _____

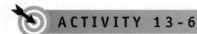

ACTIVITY 13-6

TRANSCRIBE INTRAVENOUS MEDICATION ORDERS

Materials Needed   Black ink pen

Red ink pen (depending on hospital policy)

Physicians' Desk Reference or pharmacology reference material

Medication time schedule (Table 13-2 in *LaFleur Brooks' Health Unit Coordinating,* 7th edition)

MAR used in Activity 13-5

Computer and Practice Activity Software for Transcription of Physicians' Orders

Directions

Refer to Physicians' Order Sheet 13-6 in your patient's chart. Practice transcribing the intravenous (IV) medication orders by performing the following steps. Check with your instructor for variations of the procedure to adapt it to the practice in your area. Place a check mark (✓) in the box as you complete each step.

Steps for Transcribing Intravenous Medication Orders

1. Read the orders. ☐

2. Obtain the MAR. ☐

3. Order medications by faxing or sending the pharmacy copy of the doctor's orders to the pharmacy. ☐

> ### ★ HIGH PRIORITY
>
> An admixture is a medication added to 500 to 1000 mL of IV solution; a piggyback medication that is usually administered intravenously in 50 to 100 mL of fluid. A bolus or IV push is a medication administered intravenously but not added to an IV solution.

4. Write "faxed pc" or "pcs" with the time and your initials in ink on the doctor's order sheet to indicate that the pharmacy copy has been sent. ☐

5. Enter medications on your patient's medication profile by using a computer and the practice software by:

　a. typing in (1) today's date; (2) the name of the medication and dosage; (3) the route; (4) the frequency; (5) and the qualifying phrase, if used ☐

OR

Document the medications in ink on the MAR under the correct heading (standing, prn, stat, etc.) by:

　a. writing (1) today's date; (2) the name of the medication and dosage; (3) the route; (4) the frequency; (5) and the qualifying phrase, if used ☐

> ### ★ HIGH PRIORITY
>
> In transcribing admixture orders, practice varies regarding whether the IV solution is documented on the MAR.

　b. writing "m" in ink in the symbol column in front of the order on the doctor's order sheet to indicate completion of the documentation ☐

6. Recheck each step for accuracy. ☐

7. Sign off the orders to indicate completion of transcription. ☐

Place a check mark (✓) in the following box to indicate that you have completed Activity 13-6.

☐ Transcribe Intravenous Medication Orders   Date: _____

ACTIVITY 13-7

TRANSCRIBE MEDICATION ORDERS WITH AUTOMATIC STOP DATES

Materials Needed   Black ink pen

Red ink pen (depending on hospital policy)

Physicians' Desk Reference or pharmacology reference material

Medication time schedule (Table 13-2 in *LaFleur Brooks' Health Unit Coordinating,* 7th edition)

MAR used in Activity 13-6

Computer and Practice Activity Software for Transcription of Physicians' Orders

Directions

Refer to Physicians' Order Sheet 13-7 in your patient's chart. Practice transcribing the medication orders by performing the following steps. Check with your instructor for variations of the procedure to adapt it to the practice in your area. Place a check mark (✓) in the box as you complete each step.

Steps for Transcribing Medication Orders with Automatic Stop Dates

1. Read the orders.   ☐

2. Obtain the MAR.   ☐

3. Order medications by faxing or sending the pharmacy copy of the doctor's orders to the pharmacy.   ☐

4. Write "faxed pc" or "pcs" with the time and your initials in ink on the doctor's order sheet to indicate that the pharmacy copy has been sent.   ☐

⭐ HIGH PRIORITY

Medications such as narcotics, sedatives, antibiotics, and anticoagulants have automatic stop dates. The physician will either reorder the medication or discontinue it on a stamped or written request on the physicians' order sheet. (The HUC or the nurse is responsible for placing this request on the order sheet.) Check with your instructor for the medications that have automatic stop dates in your area.

---

5. Enter medications on your patient's medication profile by using a computer and the practice software by:

    a. typing in (1) today's date; (2) the name of the medication and dosage; (3) the route; (4) the frequency; (5) and the qualifying phrase, if used   ☐

OR

Document the medications in ink on the MAR under the correct heading (standing, prn, stat, etc.) by:

    a. writing (1) today's date; (2) the name of the medication and dosage; (3) the route; (4) the frequency; (5) and the qualifying phrase, if used   ☐

★ **HIGH PRIORITY**

If two doses are included in one medication order, the doses may need to be written on separate lines on the MAR.

Example:

Acetaminophen 1 or 2 caps. PO q3-4h prn

Date	Drug	Dose	Route	Schedule
0/00	acetaminophen	1 cap	PO	3-4 h prn
0/00	acetaminophen	2 caps	PO	3-4 h prn

   b. writing "m" in ink in the symbol column in front of the order on the physicians' order sheet to indicate completion of the documentation ☐

6. Recheck each step for accuracy. ☐

7. Sign off the orders to indicate completion of transcription. ☐

Place a check mark (✓) in the following box to indicate that you have completed Activity 13-7.

☐ Transcribe Medication Orders with Automatic Stop Dates   Date: _____

◎ **ACTIVITY 13-8**

TRANSCRIBE ORDERS TO RENEW MEDICATIONS THAT HAVE AUTOMATIC STOP DATES

Materials Needed   Black ink pen

                                 Red ink pen (depending on hospital policy)

                                 Physicians' Desk Reference or pharmacology reference material

                                 MAR used in Activity 13-7

                                 Computer and Practice Activity Software for Transcription of Physicians' Orders

Directions

Refer to Physicians' Order Sheet 13-8 in your patient's chart. Practice transcribing the orders to renew the medications by performing the following steps. Check with your instructor for variations of the procedure to adapt it to the practice in your area. Place a check mark (✓) in the box as you complete each step.

Steps for Transcribing Orders to Renew Medications That Have Automatic Stop Dates

1. Read the orders. ☐

2. Obtain the MAR. ☐

3. Notify the pharmacy department that the medications have been renewed by:
   a. faxing or sending the pharmacy copy of the doctor's order sheet to the pharmacy ☐
   b. writing "faxed pc" or "pcs" with the time and your initials in ink on the doctor's order sheet to indicate that the pharmacy copy has been sent ☐

4. Renew the medications on the MAR by:
   a. placing a slash mark across the stop date in the stop date column ☐
   b. writing the new stop date in ink near the stop date column next to the medication ☐

★ **HIGH PRIORITY**

> The method of renewing medication on the MAR may vary among hospitals. In some hospitals, the stop date is written in pencil and is erased and a new stop date is entered (the original order date remains and is written in ink).

    c. writing "m" in ink in the symbol column in front of the order on the doctor's order sheet to indicate completion of the documentation ☐

OR

Enter the new stop dates on your patient's medication profile by using a computer and the practice software ☐

5. Recheck each step for accuracy. ☐

6. Sign off the order to indicate completion of transcription. ☐

Place a check mark (✓) in the following box to indicate that you have completed Activity 13-8.

☐ Transcribe Orders to Renew Medications
That Have Automatic Stop Dates   Date: _____

◎ **ACTIVITY 13-9**

TRANSCRIBE ORDERS TO DISCONTINUE MEDICATIONS

Materials Needed   Black ink pen
                            Yellow highlighter
                            MAR used in Activity 13-8
                            Computer and Practice Activity Software for Transcription of Physicians' Orders

Directions

Refer to Physicians' Order Sheet 13-9 in your patient's chart. Practice transcribing orders to discontinue the medications by performing the following steps. Check with your instructor for variations of the procedure to adapt it to the practice in your area. Place a check mark (✓) in the box as you complete each step.

Steps for Transcribing Orders to Discontinue Medications

1. Read the orders. ☐

2. Obtain the MAR. ☐

3. Notify the pharmacy department that the medications have been discontinued by:
    a. faxing or sending the pharmacy copy of the doctor's order sheet to the pharmacy ☐
    b. writing "faxed pc" or "pcs" with the time and your initials in ink on the doctor's order sheet to indicate that the pharmacy copy has been sent ☐

4. Discontinue the medications on the MAR by:
    a. highlighting the medication and all spaces on the line of the discontinued medication using a yellow highlighter ☐
    b. writing "D/C" in ink on the line of the discontinued medication under the correct date ☐
    c. writing "m" in ink in the symbol column in front of the order on the doctor's order sheet to indicate completion of the documentation ☐

OR

Discontinue the medications on your patient's medication profile by typing the discontinue date in the DC date field by using a computer and the practice software ☐

5. Recheck each step for accuracy. ☐

6. Sign off the orders to indicate completion of transcription. ☐

Place a check mark (✓) in the following box to indicate that you have completed Activity 13-9.

☐ Transcribe Orders to Discontinue Medications   Date: _____

◎ ACTIVITY 13-10

TRANSCRIBE ORDERS FOR MEDICATION CHANGES

Materials Needed   Black ink pen

Red ink pen (depending on hospital policy)

Yellow highlighter

Medication time schedule (Table 13-2 in *LaFleur Brooks' Health Unit Coordinating,* 7th edition)

MAR used in Activity 13-9

Computer and Practice Activity Software for Transcription of Physicians' Orders

Directions

Refer to Physicians' Order Sheet 13-10 in your patient's chart. Practice transcribing the orders for the medication changes by performing the following steps. Check with your instructor for variations of the procedure to adapt it to the practice in your area. Place a check mark (✓) in the box as you complete each step.

Steps for Transcribing Orders for Medication Changes

1. Read the orders.   ☐
2. Obtain the MAR.   ☐
3. Notify the pharmacy department that the medications have been changed by:
   a. faxing or sending the pharmacy copy of the doctor's order sheet to the pharmacy   ☐
   b. writing "faxed pc" or "pcs" with the time and your initials in ink on the doctor's order sheet to
      indicate that the pharmacy copy has been sent   ☐
4. Document the medication changes on the MAR by:
   a. highlighting the original order and the unused spaces using the yellow highlighter   ☐
   b. writing "D/C" or "D" in ink on the line of the discontinued or changed medication under the
      correct date   ☐
   c. writing in the new order on a new line   ☐
   d. writing "m" in ink in the symbol column in front of the order on the doctor's order sheet to
      indicate completion of the documentation   ☐

OR

Document the medication change on your patient's medication profile by typing "DC'd" next to the discontinued
medication and then typing the correct medication on the next line by using a computer and the practice software   ☐

5. Recheck each step for accuracy.   ☐
6. Sign off the orders to indicate completion of transcription.   ☐

Place a check mark (✓) in the following box to indicate that you have completed Activity 13-10.

☐ Transcribe Orders for Medication Changes   Date: _____

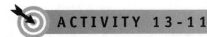

TRANSCRIBE A REVIEW SET OF MEDICATION ORDERS

Materials Needed   Black ink pen

Red ink pen (depending on hospital policy)

Yellow highlighter

Physicians' Desk Reference or pharmacology reference material

Medication time schedule (Table 13-2 in *LaFleur Brooks' Health Unit Coordinating,* 7th edition)

MAR used in Activity 13-10

Computer and Practice Activity Software for Transcription of Physicians' Orders

Directions

Refer to Physicians' Order Sheet 13-11 in your patient's chart. Transcribe the orders. They include changing, renewing, and discontinuing medication orders. Refer to previous activities for the appropriate transcription steps as needed.

Steps for Transcribing a Review Set of Medication Orders

1. Read the orders.   ❑

2. Order medications by faxing or sending the pharmacy copy of the doctor's orders to the pharmacy
and write "faxed pc" or "pcs" with the time and your initials in ink on the doctor's order sheet.   ❑

3. Check for any stat orders.   ❑

4. Obtain the MAR.   ❑

5. Order any supplies needed.   ❑

6. Document the medications on the MAR   ❑

OR

Enter the medications on your patient's medication profile by using a computer and the practice software   ❑

7. Recheck each step for accuracy.   ❑

8. Sign off the orders to indicate completion of transcription.   ❑

Place a check mark (✓) in the following box to indicate that you have completed Activity 13-11.

❑ Transcribe a Review Set of Medication Orders   Date: _____

 ACTIVITY 13-12

TRANSCRIBE A REVIEW SET OF DOCTORS' ORDERS

Materials Needed   Black ink pen

Red ink pen (depending on hospital policy)

Pencil

Eraser

Patient's ID labels (if using requisition method)

Necessary requisition forms (if using requisition method)

Physicians' Desk Reference or pharmacology reference material

Medication time schedule (Table 13-2 in *LaFleur Brooks' Health Unit Coordinating,* 7th edition)

Kardex form used in previous chapters

MAR used in Activity 13-11

Computer and Practice Activity Software for Transcription of Physicians' Orders

Directions

Refer to Physicians' Order Sheet 13-12 in your patient's chart. Transcribe the orders. Refer to the previous activities for the appropriate transcription steps as needed.

Steps for Transcribing a Review Set of Doctors' Orders

1. Read the orders. ❏
2. Order medications by faxing or sending the pharmacy copy of the doctors' orders to the pharmacy and write "faxed pc" or "pcs" with the time and your initials in ink on the doctor's order sheet. ❏
3. Check for any stat orders. ❏
4. Make any necessary phone calls. ❏
5. Obtain the necessary forms. ❏

Suggestion to the student: Use this space to list the forms you will need.

6. Order as necessary. ❏
7. Document the orders on the Kardex form. ❏
8. Document the medications on the MAR ❏

OR

Enter the medications on your patient's medication profile by using a computer and the practice software. ❏

9. Recheck each step for accuracy. ❏
10. Sign off the orders to indicate completion of transcription. ❏

★ HIGH PRIORITY

Transcribing doctors' orders is a critical task, and an error could cause harm to a patient. If not absolutely sure about the medication or if you have any doubt about an order, ask the patient's nurse or the doctor who wrote the order.

Place a check mark (✓) in the following box to indicate that you have completed Activity 13-12.

❏ Transcribe a Review Set of Doctors' Orders   Date: _____

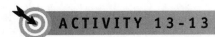

LOCATE MEDICATIONS IN THE *PHYSICIANS' DESK REFERENCE*

Materials Needed Pen or pencil

Physicians' Desk Reference or pharmacology reference material

Paper

Directions

Locate the following medications in the *Physicians' Desk Reference, Nursing Drug Reference,* or other reference material, and briefly state the purpose of each. Your instructor may ask you to locate and provide additional information. Perform the following steps. Place a check mark (✓) in the box as you complete each step.

Medications

Dilantin	Synthroid	Lasix	Allegra	Demerol
flurazepam	ibuprofen	alprazolam	heparin	oxycodone

Steps for Locating Medications in the Physicians' Desk Reference

1. Locate the medication (listed alphabetically) in the "Generic and Brand Name Index" (pink section) of the *Physicians' Desk Reference*. ❑

2. Turn to the page (higher number) indicated next to the medication. ❑

3. Read the paragraphs titled "Indications and Usage" under drug name and write the purpose of the medication. ❑

Place a check mark (✓) in the following box to indicate that you have completed Activity 13-13.

❑ Locate Medications in the *Physicians' Desk Reference*   Date: _____

TRANSCRIBE RECORDED TELEPHONE MESSAGES

Materials Needed Pen or pencil

Note pad

Directions

Practice transcribing the following printed telephone messages by performing the following steps. Place a check mark (✓) in the box as you complete each step.

Telephone Messages

1. "This is Dr. Joan Peters. Would you let Francine Pack's nurse know that I will be in to write TPN orders in about a half an hour?"

2. "This is Dave in the pharmacy. I received a pharmacy copy that was not labeled with a patient's name. I am sending it back to you to identify, label, and send back to me."

3. "This is Dr. Hy Hopes. Would you please call Dr. Thomas Ryan and remind him of the consult I requested on James Brown Tuesday morning?"

Steps for Transcribing Telephone Messages

1. Have someone read these messages to you while you transcribe them on a note pad. ☐

2. Write down for whom the message is intended. ☐

3. Write down the caller's name. ☐

4. Write down the date and time of the call. ☐

5. Write down the purpose of the call. ☐

6. If a return call is expected, write down the number to call. ☐

7. Sign your name to the message. ☐

Place a check mark (✓) in the following box to indicate that you have completed Activity 13-15.

☐ Record Telephone Messages   Date: _____

PHYSICIANS' ORDER SHEET 13-1

DATE	TIME	SYMBOL	ORDERS
02/19	0700	M	Allergy to morphine sulfate
		M	Coreg 25 mg PO bid
		M	Aldactone 50 mg PO q day
PC sent 0710		M	glimepiride 2 mg PO q day
DC'd		M	furosemide 20 mg PO bid
		M	Lipitor 10 mg PO qhs
			Dr. Smith-Jones
			feb.19/19, 0710. J. Rviz, HUC

PHYSICIANS' ORDER SHEET 13-2

DATE	TIME	SYMBOL	ORDERS
02/20	0700	M	compazine supp 25 mg. PR q 12 hr N/V
		M	ibuprofen 600 mg PO tid with food PRN mild pain
DC sent	0710	M	lorazepam 0.5 mg PO qh for agitation or anxiety
			Dr. Smith-Jones
			feb. 20/19, 0710, J. Ruiz, HUC

PHYSICIANS' ORDER SHEET 13-3

DATE	TIME	SYMBOL	ORDERS
02/21	0700	M	Singulair 10 mg PO today
		M	meperidine HCL 100 mg IM prior to drsg Δ in am
PC sent 0710		M	PPD ID lt forearm today
			Dr. Smith-Jones
			feb 20/19, 0710, J. Ruiz HUC

PHYSICIANS' ORDER SHEET 13-4 *Short series.*

DATE.	TIME	SYMBOL	ORDERS
02/22	0700	M	Medrol 12 mg PO bid today, then 8 mg PO bid X2d, then D/C
	PC sent	M	K-lyte 1 tablet in ½ glass H$_2$O c̄ meals X 3 days
			Dr. Smith, Jones
			Feb 22/19, 0710, J. Ruiz, HUC

PHYSICIANS' ORDER SHEET 13-5 *One time.*

DATE	TIME	SYMBOL	ORDERS
02/23	0700	M	Amiodarone 300 mg IV push now
PC sent	0710	M	Lovenox 40 mg sq stat
	Not. Mary 0710		Dr.
			Feb. 23/19, 0710, J. Ruiz, HUC

PHYSICIANS' ORDER SHEET 13-6 *standing.*

DATE	TIME	SYMBOL	ORDERS
02/24	0700	M PC sent	Ambien 10 mg PO q hs
		M PC sent	oxycodone 5 mg PO q 4-6 hr for pain
	PC sent		Dr.
			Feb. 24/19, 0710, J. Ruiz HUC

5days Antibiotic PHYSICIANS' ORDER SHEET 13-7 IV

DATE	TIME	SYMBOL	ORDERS
02/25	0700	M	ciprofloxacin 500 mg IVPB q6h *piggie bag*
		✗	Δ PICC IVF to 1000 mL D5LR c̄ 20 mEq KCl @ 100 mL/hr
PC sent	0710		Dr.
			Feb. 25/19, 0710, J. Ruiz, HUC

PHYSICIANS' ORDER SHEET 13-8 *renew*

DATE	TIME	SYMBOL	ORDERS
02/26	0700	M, present	Doctor, the following medications have expired.
present 0700		M, present	Renew:
	0710.		oxycodone 3days yes ✓ no ___
			Ambien 5days yes ✓ no ___
			Dr.
			Feb. 26/20, 0710, C. De Santis, HUC.

PHYSICIANS' ORDER SHEET 13-9 *discont.*

DATE	TIME	SYMBOL	ORDERS
02/27	0700	M	D/C glimepiride
present	0710	M	D/C lorazepam
			Dr.
			feb. 27/19, 0710, J. Rviz, HUC

PHYSICIANS' ORDER SHEET 13-10 *change (redpen)*

DATE	TIME	SYMBOL	ORDERS
			change
02/28	0700	M	Δ Lipitor to 20 mg
		M	Δ ciprofloxacin to 250 mg PO
PC sent.			Dr.
			Feb. 28/2020, 0730, C De Santis, HUC.

PHYSICIANS' ORDER SHEET 13-11

DATE	TIME	SYMBOL	ORDERS
02/29		M	Plavix 75 mg PO q day
		M	ASA 81 mg q day
			Dr.
		M, PCsent	D/C Ambien
		M	temazepam 30 mg PO q HS
		M	warfarin 5 mg PO qod
			Dr.
		M	NTG spray 0.4 mg/dose @ BS
		M	Vancomycin 10 mg/kg IVPB q6h
		M	Lidocaine bolus 100 mg IV push prn multifocal PVCs or 6 PVCs
			per min
		K	DC PICC
		K	Insert HL c̄ rout saline flushes (Kardexing)
			Dr.
			Feb 29/2020, 0800, C. De Santis, HUC

(left margin, written vertically: PC sent)

PHYSICIANS' ORDER SHEET 13-12

DATE	TIME	SYMBOL	ORDERS
			DC pneumatic comp.
			Cont wearing ted hose
			Δ atorvastatin to 40 mg PO qhs
			glyburide 2.5 or 5 mg PO qd
			hydrocortisone cm to rash on hand bid
			D/C Aldactone
			D/C ibuprofen
			Dr.

CHAPTER 14

Laboratory Orders and Recording Telephoned Laboratory Results

Activities in this Chapter:

⭐ HIGH PRIORITY

When an electronic medical record (EMR) with computerized physician order entry system has been implemented, the doctor will enter orders directly into the patient's EMR. The orders will automatically be sent to the laboratory department. The HUC may be responsible for instructing or assisting the physician or nurse in requisitioning the laboratory tests. The HUC may also be the primary communicator between the physician, the nursing staff, and the laboratory personnel about laboratory tests. Effective communication about stat and timed laboratory draws and test results may be a primary responsibility of the HUC on any nursing unit. The paper-based requisition method is included for learning purposes.

★ **HIGH PRIORITY**

Review Chapter 14 in *LaFleur Brooks' Health Unit Coordinating*, 7th edition, for explanations of doctors' orders, laboratory tests, and definitions of abbreviations.

Place the Physicians' Order Sheets located at the end of this chapter in your patient's chart. Follow the directions for each activity to transcribe orders.

 ACTIVITY 14-1

TRANSCRIBE HEMATOLOGY/COAGULATION ORDERS

Materials Needed
Black ink pen
Red ink pen (depending on hospital policy)
Pencil
Eraser
Kardex form used in previous chapters
Patient ID labels (if using requisition method)
Laboratory requisition form (if using requisition method)
Computer and Practice Activity Software for Transcription of Physicians' Orders

Directions

Refer to Physicians' Order Sheet 14-1 (obtained from the end of this chapter) in your patient's chart. Practice transcribing the hematology/coagulation orders by performing the following steps. Check with your instructor for variations of the procedure to adapt it to the practice in your area. Place a check mark (✓) in the box as you complete each step.

Steps for Transcribing Hematology/Coagulation Orders

1. Read the orders. ❏

2. Obtain the Kardex form and requisition form if using the requisition method. ❏

3. Order the tests from the laboratory department. ❏

Use the computer and practice software by:
  a. selecting Enter Orders on the home screen ❏
  b. selecting the patient's name from the census on the viewing screen ❏
  c. selecting the laboratory department from the department menu on the viewing screen ❏
  d. selecting the hematology division from the laboratory department viewing screen ❏
  e. typing in the pertinent information ❏
  f. selecting the tests to be ordered from the menu on the viewing screen ❏
  g. writing "ord" in ink above each order on the doctor's order sheet to indicate that the test has been ordered ❏

★ **HIGH PRIORITY**

In the hospital setting, writing "ord" or the computer order number above each laboratory test ordered will reduce the risk of missing an order.

  h. sending the order by pressing Enter Order(s) on the viewing screen ❏

Use the requisition form by:
   a. affixing the patient's ID label to the form
   b. writing in the pertinent information
   c. placing a check mark (✓) in the column next to the tests to be ordered
   d. writing "ord" in ink above each order on the doctor's order sheet to indicate that the test has been ordered
   e. sending the requisition

4. Document the orders by:
   a. writing the date and the order in pencil in the laboratory column on the Kardex form
   b. writing "K" in ink in the symbol column in front of the order on the doctor's order sheet to indicate completion of the documentation

5. Recheck each step for accuracy.

6. Sign off the orders to indicate completion of transcription.

Place a check mark (✓) in the following box to indicate that you have completed Activity 14-1.

❏ Transcribe Hematology/Coagulation Orders   Date: _____

✦ ACTIVITY 14-2

TRANSCRIBE DAILY LABORATORY ORDERS

Materials Needed   Black ink pen

Red ink pen (depending on hospital policy)

Pencil

Eraser

Kardex form used in Activity 14-1

Patient ID labels (if using requisition method)

Laboratory requisition form (if using requisition method)

Computer and Practice Activity Software for Transcription of Physicians' Orders

Directions

Refer to Physicians' Order Sheet 14-2 in your patient's chart. Practice transcribing the daily laboratory orders by performing the following steps. Check with your instructor for variations of the procedure to adapt it to the practice in your area. Place a check mark (✓) in the box as you complete each step.

Steps for Transcribing Daily Laboratory Orders

1. Read the orders.   ❏

★ HIGH PRIORITY

The date and time that the daily laboratory tests will be drawn vary according to hospital policy, and may even vary from unit to unit in the same hospital. Most daily laboratory tests are ordered to be done at 0400 so physicians may have the results when they make rounds. Check with your instructor for the practice in your area.

2. Obtain the Kardex form and requisition form if using the requisition method.   ❏

3. Order the tests from the laboratory department.   ❏

Use the computer and practice software by:
a. selecting Enter Orders on the home screen ☐
b. selecting the patient's name from the census on the viewing screen ☐
c. selecting the laboratory department from the department menu on the viewing screen ☐
d. selecting the hematology division from the laboratory department viewing screen ☐
e. typing in the pertinent information ☐
f. selecting the tests to be ordered from the menu on the viewing screen ☐
g. writing "ord" in ink above each order on the doctor's order sheet to indicate that the test has been ordered ☐
h. sending the order by pressing Enter Order(s) on the viewing screen ☐

Use the requisition form by:
a. affixing the patient's ID label to the form ☐
b. writing in the pertinent information ☐
c. placing a check mark (✓) in the column next to the tests to be ordered ☐
d. writing "ord" in ink above each order on the doctor's order sheet to indicate that the test has been ordered ☐
e. sending the requisition ☐

4. Document the orders by:
a. writing the date and the order in pencil in the daily laboratory column on the Kardex form ☐
b. writing "K" in ink in the symbol column in front of the order on the doctor's order sheet to indicate completion of the documentation ☐

5. Recheck each step for accuracy. ☐

6. Sign off the orders to indicate completion of transcription. ☐

★ **HIGH PRIORITY**

Daily laboratory tests may be ordered from all divisions of the laboratory. Most computer systems can order daily diagnostic tests several days in advance. If not, the daily order must be entered each day for the following day.

Place a check mark (✓) in the following box to indicate that you have completed Activity 14-2.

☐ Transcribe Daily Laboratory Orders

Date: _____

◎ **ACTIVITY 14-3**

TRANSCRIBE CHEMISTRY ORDERS

Materials Needed

Black ink pen
Red ink pen (depending on hospital policy)
Pencil
Eraser
Kardex form used in Activity 14-2
Patient ID labels (if using requisition method)
Laboratory requisition form (if using requisition method)
Computer and Practice Activity Software for Transcription of Physicians' Orders

Directions

Refer to Physicians' Order Sheet 14-3 in your patient's chart. Practice transcribing the chemistry orders by performing the following steps. Check with your instructor for variations of the procedure to adapt it to the practice in your area. Place a check mark (✓) in the box as you complete each step.

Steps for Transcribing Chemistry Orders

1. Read the orders. ❑

2. Obtain the Kardex form and requisition form if using the requisition method. ❑

3. Order the tests from the laboratory department. ❑

Use the computer and practice software by:
   a. selecting Enter Orders from the home screen ❑
   b. selecting the patient's name from the census on the viewing screen ❑
   c. selecting the laboratory department from the department menu on the viewing screen ❑
   d. selecting the chemistry division from the laboratory department viewing screen ❑
   e. typing in the pertinent information ❑
   f. selecting the tests to be ordered from the menu on the viewing screen ❑
   g. writing "ord" in ink above each order on the doctor's order sheet to indicate that the test has been ordered ❑
   h. sending the order by pressing Enter Order(s) on the viewing screen ❑

Use the requisition form by:
   a. affixing the patient's ID label to the form ❑
   b. writing in the pertinent information ❑
   c. placing a check mark (✓) in the column next to the tests to be ordered ❑
   d. writing "ord" in ink above each order on the doctor's order sheet to indicate that the test has been ordered ❑
   e. sending the requisition ❑

4. Document the orders by:
   a. writing the date and the order in pencil in the laboratory column on the Kardex form ❑
   b. writing "K" in ink in the symbol column in front of the order on the doctor's order sheet to indicate completion of the documentation ❑

5. Recheck each step for accuracy. ❑

6. Sign off the orders to indicate completion of transcription. ❑

Place a check mark (✓) in the following box to indicate that you have completed Activity 14-3.

❑ Transcribe Chemistry Orders   Date: _____

ACTIVITY 14-4

TRANSCRIBE STAT LABORATORY ORDERS

Materials Needed   Black ink pen
Red ink pen (depending on hospital policy)
Pencil
Eraser
Kardex form used in Activity 14-3
Patient ID labels (if using requisition method)
Laboratory requisition form (if using requisition method)
Computer and Practice Activity Software for Transcription of Physicians' Orders

Directions

Refer to Physicians' Order Sheet 14-4 in your patient's chart. Practice transcribing the stat laboratory orders by performing the following steps. Check with your instructor for variations of the procedure to adapt it to the practice in your area. Place a check mark (✓) in the box as you complete each step.

Steps for Transcribing Stat Laboratory Orders

1. Read the orders.   ❑

> ⭐ **HIGH PRIORITY**
>
> Communicate stat laboratory orders by immediately notifying the laboratory or nursing personnel responsible for carrying out the order. Include the name of the patient, the room number, and the test requested; if nursing personnel will be drawing the laboratory specimen, provide a copy of the order. Write the word "notified" and the time next to the stat order on the doctor's order sheet. Stat orders communicated by computer may not require a telephone call to laboratory personnel; enter "stat" in the correct information field. Notify the laboratory or nursing personnel if there are additional laboratory tests to be done on a routine or random basis that may be done on the specimen drawn for the stat order.

2. Notify the clinical laboratory by placing a telephone call to the appropriate department. Document the phone call on the doctor's order sheet.   ❑

3. Obtain the Kardex form and requisition form if using the requisition method.   ❑

4. Order the tests from the laboratory department.   ❑

Use the computer and practice software by:
  a. selecting Enter Orders from the home screen   ❑
  b. selecting the patient's name from the census on the viewing screen   ❑
  c. selecting the laboratory department from the department menu on the viewing screen   ❑
  d. selecting the appropriate division from the laboratory department viewing screen   ❑
  e. typing in the pertinent information (remember to select "stat" on the computer)   ❑
  f. selecting the tests to be ordered from the menu on the viewing screen   ❑
  g. writing "ord" in ink above each order on the doctor's order sheet to indicate that the test has been ordered   ❑
  h. sending the order by pressing Enter Order(s) on the viewing screen   ❑

Use the requisition form by:
  a. affixing the patient's ID label to the form   ❑
  b. writing in the pertinent information   ❑
  c. placing a check mark (✓) in the column next to the tests to be ordered   ❑
  d. writing "ord" in ink above each order on the doctor's order sheet to indicate that the test has been ordered   ❑
  e. sending the requisition   ❑

4. Document the orders by:
  a. writing the date and order in pencil in the laboratory column on the Kardex form   ❑
  b. writing "K" in ink in the symbol column in front of the order on the doctor's order sheet to indicate completion of the documentation   ❑

5. Recheck each step for accuracy.   ❑

6. Sign off the order to indicate completion of transcription.   ❑

Place a check mark (✓) in the following box to indicate that you have completed Activity 14-4.

❑ Transcribe Stat Laboratory Orders   Date: _____

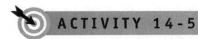 **ACTIVITY 14-5**

TRANSCRIBE FASTING AND NPO LABORATORY ORDERS

Materials Needed   Black ink pen

Red ink pen (depending on hospital policy)

Pencil

Eraser

Kardex form used in Activity 14-4

Patient ID labels (if using requisition method)

Laboratory requisition form (if using requisition method)

Computer and Practice Activity Software for Transcription of Physicians' Orders

Fasting and nothing-by-mouth (NPO) list for laboratory studies (Table 14-2 in *LaFleur Brooks' Health Unit Coordinating,* 7th edition)

Directions

Refer to Physicians' Order Sheet 14-5 in your patient's chart. Practice transcribing the fasting and NPO laboratory orders by performing the following steps. Check with your instructor for variations of the procedure to adapt it to the practice in your area. Place a check mark (✓) in the box as you complete each step.

Steps for Transcribing Fasting and NPO Laboratory Orders

1. Read the orders.   ☐

2. Obtain the Kardex form and requisition form if using the requisition method.   ☐

3. Order the tests from the laboratory department.   ☐

Use the computer and practice software by:

 a. selecting Enter Order on the home screen   ☐

 b. selecting the patient's name from the census on the viewing screen   ☐

 c. selecting the laboratory department from the department menu on the viewing screen   ☐

 d. selecting the chemistry division from the laboratory department viewing screen   ☐

 e. typing in the pertinent information   ☐

 f. selecting the tests to be ordered from the menu on the viewing screen   ☐

 g. writing "ord" in ink above each order on the doctor's order sheet to indicate that the test has been ordered   ☐

 h. sending the order by pressing Enter Order(s) on the viewing screen   ☐

Use the requisition form by:

 a. affixing the patient's ID label to the form   ☐

 b. writing in the pertinent information   ☐

 c. placing a check mark (✓) in the column next to the tests to be ordered   ☐

 d. writing "ord" in ink above each order on the doctor's order sheet to indicate that the test has been ordered   ☐

 e. sending the requisition   ☐

★ HIGH PRIORITY

Select or enter the date and time personnel should draw the blood when ordering a laboratory test on the computer. If the test is routine, it is not necessary to select or enter a time because it will be collected with the next routine laboratory draw (usually within 2 hours). When using the requisition method, if necessary write the date and time to draw the blood at the top of the requisition form. For fasting and NPO orders, the blood is drawn before breakfast the following day. You may need to enter the time for the routine morning blood draw, such as "0430."

---

4. Document the orders by:
   a. writing the date and order in pencil in the laboratory column on the Kardex form   ❑
   b. writing "K" in ink in the symbol column in front of the order on the doctor's order sheet to indicate completion of the documentation   ❑

5. Recheck each step for accuracy.   ❑

6. Sign off the orders to indicate completion of transcription.   ❑

Place a check mark (✓) in the following box to indicate that you have completed Activity 14-5.

❑ Transcribe Fasting and NPO Laboratory Orders   Date: _____

◎ ACTIVITY 14-6

TRANSCRIBE A REVIEW SET OF LABORATORY ORDERS

Materials Needed
Black ink pen
Red ink pen (depending on hospital policy)
Pencil
Eraser
Kardex form used in Activity 14-5
Patient ID labels (if using requisition method)
Laboratory requisition forms (if using requisition method)
Computer and Practice Activity Software for Transcription of Physicians' Orders
Fasting and NPO lists for laboratory studies (Table 14-6)

Directions

Refer to Physicians' Order Sheet 14-6 in your patient's chart. Transcribe the orders, which include hematology/coagulation, daily laboratory studies, chemistry, toxicology, stat, and fasting and NPO laboratory orders. Refer to previous activities for the appropriate transcription steps as needed.

★ HIGH PRIORITY

Peak-and-trough drug level tests are ordered from the toxicology division of the laboratory and require the HUC to coordinate the drawing of the blood with the nurse administering the drug, such as vancomycin. The tests are ordered "timed," meaning that they will be drawn at the specific time indicated.

Steps for Transcribing a Review Set of Laboratory Orders

1. Read the orders.   ❑
2. Check orders for stats.   ❑
3. Place and document telephone call for notification of stats.   ❑
4. Obtain the Kardex form and requisition forms if using the requisition method.   ❑
5. Order the tests.   ❑
6. Document the orders on the Kardex form.   ❑
7. Recheck each step for accuracy.   ❑
8. Sign off the orders to indicate completion of transcription.   ❑

Place a check mark (✓) in the following box to indicate that you have completed Activity 14-6.

☐ Transcribe a Review Set of Laboratory Orders   Date: _____

⊙ ACTIVITY 14-7

TRANSCRIBE MICROBIOLOGY/BACTERIOLOGY ORDERS

Materials Needed   Black ink pen

Red ink pen (depending on hospital policy)

Pencil

Eraser

Kardex form used in Activity 14-6

Patient ID labels (if using requisition method)

Laboratory requisition form (if using requisition method)

Computer and Practice Activity Software for Transcription of Physicians' Orders

Directions

Refer to Physicians' Order Sheet 14-7 in your patient's chart. Practice transcribing the microbiology/bacteriology orders by performing the following steps. Check with your instructor for variations of the procedure to adapt it to the practice in your area. Place a check mark (✓) in the box as you complete each step.

★ HIGH PRIORITY

Standard precautions require that all specimens be bagged and labeled with patient ID information. The person collecting the specimen should write his or her initials and the date and time that the specimen was collected on the patient ID label. In emergency situations, the HUC may need to label and bag specimens. The HUC should keep gloves in a drawer at the nursing station to wear when handling collected specimens (bagged or not) and should wash his or her hands after handling specimens, even if bagged.

Steps for Transcribing Microbiology/Bacteriology Orders

1. Read the orders.   ☐

2. Obtain the Kardex form and requisition forms if using the requisition method.   ☐

3. Order the tests from the laboratory department.   ☐

Use the computer and practice software by:

  a. selecting Enter Orders on the home screen   ☐

  b. selecting the patient's name from the census on the viewing screen   ☐

  c. selecting the laboratory department from the department menu on the viewing screen   ☐

  d. selecting the microbiology division from the laboratory department viewing screen   ☐

  e. typing in the pertinent information, including the name(s) of any antibiotic medication
     the patient is on.   ☐

  f. selecting the specimen source from the menu on the viewing screen   ☐

  g. selecting the tests to be performed from the menu on the viewing screen   ☐

> ⭐ **HIGH PRIORITY**
>
> When filling out the requisition for a microbiology test, the HUC may need to identify whether the patient is currently on antibiotic medication. This information is entered on the requisition.

 h. writing "ord" in ink above each order on the doctor's order sheet to indicate that the test has been ordered ☐

 i. when collected, looking through the bag that contains the specimen and checking the label on the specimen for proper patient ID, date, and time collected, and for the initials of the person who collected the specimen ☐

> ⭐ **HIGH PRIORITY**
>
> The order is usually entered into the computer when the specimen is obtained. The bagged, labeled specimen is then sent to the laboratory with a copy of the information entered into the computer.

 j. sending the specimen with a copy of the order to the laboratory ☐

> ⭐ **HIGH PRIORITY**
>
> Each specimen obtained from the patient by the nurse requires a separate requisition and label because specimens may be collected at different times or sent to different divisions within the laboratory. In the hospital setting, the label is paper-clipped to the requisition and kept at the nursing unit in a designated area until the nurse obtains the specimen.

Use the requisition form by:
 a. affixing the patient's ID label to the form ☐
 b. writing in the pertinent information ☐
 c. placing a check mark (✓) in the column next to the tests to be ordered ☐
 d. writing "ord" in ink above each order on the doctor's order sheet to indicate that the test has been ordered ☐
 e. when collected, checking the label on the specimen for proper patient ID, date, and time collected, and for the initials of person who collected the specimen ☐
 f. sending the specimen with the requisition to the laboratory ☐

4. Document the orders by:
 a. writing the date and the order in pencil in the laboratory column on the Kardex form ☐
 b. writing "K" in ink in the symbol column in front of the order on the doctor's order sheet to indicate completion of the documentation ☐

5. Recheck each step for accuracy. ☐

6. Sign off the orders to indicate completion of transcription. ☐

Place a check mark (✓) in the following box to indicate that you have completed Activity 14-7.

☐ Transcribe Microbiology/Bacteriology Orders   Date: _____

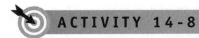

ACTIVITY 14-8

TRANSCRIBE SEROLOGY ORDERS

Materials Needed   Black ink pen
Red ink pen (depending on hospital policy)
Pencil
Eraser
Kardex form used in Activity 14-7
Patient ID labels (if using requisition method)
Laboratory requisition form (if using requisition method)
Computer and Practice Activity Software for Transcription of Physicians' Orders

Directions

Refer to Physicians' Order Sheet 14-8 in your patient's chart. Practice transcribing the serology orders by performing the following steps. Check with your instructor for variations of the procedure to adapt it to the practice in your area. Place a check mark (✓) in the box as you complete each step.

> ★ **HIGH PRIORITY**
>
> Many serology orders include the methodology by which the physician would like the serologic test to be performed. This information may be included on the computer screen or the requisition, or it may be necessary to type or write the information in the comment section.

Steps for Transcribing Serology Orders

1. Read the orders. ❑
2. Obtain the Kardex form and requisition form if using the requisition method. ❑
3. Order the tests from the laboratory department. ❑

Use the computer and practice software by:
  a. selecting Enter Orders on the home screen ❑
  b. selecting the patient's name from the census on the viewing screen ❑
  c. selecting the laboratory department from the department menu on the viewing screen ❑
  d. selecting the serology division from the laboratory department viewing screen ❑
  e. typing in the pertinent information ❑
  f. selecting the tests to be ordered from the menu on the viewing screen ❑
  g. writing "ord" in ink above each order on the doctor's order sheet to indicate that the test has been ordered ❑
  h. sending the order by pressing Enter Order(s) on the viewing screen ❑

Use the requisition form by:
  a. affixing the patient's ID label to the form ❑
  b. writing in the pertinent information ❑
  c. placing a check mark (✓) in the column next to the tests to be ordered ❑
  d. writing "ord" in ink above each order on the doctor's order sheet to indicate that the test has been ordered ❑
  e. sending the requisition ❑

4. Document the orders by:
  a. writing the date and the order in pencil in the laboratory column on the Kardex form ❑
  b. writing "K" in ink in the symbol column in front of the order on the doctor's order sheet to indicate completion of the documentation ❑

5. Recheck each step for accuracy. ❑
6. Sign off the order to indicate completion of transcription. ❑

Place a check mark (✓) in the following box to indicate that you have completed Activity 14-8.

☐ Transcribe Serology Orders   Date: _____

ACTIVITY 14-9

TRANSCRIBE A BLOOD BANK ORDER

Materials Needed   Black ink pen
                        Red ink pen (depending on hospital policy)
                        Pencil
                        Eraser
                        Kardex form used in Activity 14-8
                        Patient ID labels
                        Blood bank requisition (if using requisition method)
                        Consent for transfusions form
                        Computer and Practice Activity Software for Transcription of Physicians' Orders

Directions

Refer to Physicians' Order Sheet 14-9 in your patient's chart. Practice transcribing the blood bank order by performing the following steps. Check with your instructor for variations of the procedure to adapt it to the practice in your area. Place a check mark (✓) in the box as you complete each step.

> ★ **HIGH PRIORITY**
>
> Because receiving blood of the wrong type could cause the death of a patient, mislabeled specimens have to be discarded, and the blood will have to be redrawn to be typed and crossmatched. Before sending specimens to the laboratory, the HUC should always check the name on the computer screen and the patient ID label on the specimen against the doctor's order in the chart.

Steps for Transcribing a Blood Bank Order

1. Read the order.   ☐
2. Obtain the Kardex form, consent for transfusions form, and a requisition form if using the
   requisition method.   ☐

> ★ **HIGH PRIORITY**
>
> A signed consent form for blood or blood product transfusion is required. A patient may also sign a refusal form for blood or blood product transfusions. Refer to Chapter 8 in *LaFleur Brooks' Health Unit Coordinating*, 7th edition.

3. Order the blood component from the blood bank.   ☐

Use the computer and practice software by:

a. affixing the patient's ID label to the consent form

b. writing in the pertinent information on the consent form

c. giving the consent form to the patient's nurse for the patient to sign

d. selecting Enter Orders on the home screen

e. selecting the patient's name from the census on the viewing screen

f. selecting the laboratory department from the department menu on the viewing screen

g. selecting the blood bank division from the laboratory department viewing screen

h. typing in the pertinent information

i. selecting the blood component to be ordered from the menu on the viewing screen and entering the cross match, if ordered

j. entering the number of units to be ordered from the menu on the viewing screen

k. writing "ord" in ink above each order on the doctor's order sheet to indicate that the blood has been ordered

l. sending the order by pressing Enter Order(s) on the viewing screen

Use the requisition form by:

a. affixing the patient's ID labels to the blood bank requisition form and the consent form

b. writing in the pertinent information on the consent form

c. giving the consent form to the patient's nurse for the patient to sign

d. writing in the pertinent information on the requisition

e. placing a check mark (✓) in the box next to the blood component that has been ordered and a check mark (✓) in the box next to the cross match, if ordered

f. writing the number of units in the appropriate space

g. writing "ord" in ink above each order on the doctor's order sheet to indicate that the blood has been ordered

h. sending the requisition

4. Document the order by:

a. writing the date and the order in pencil in the laboratory column on the Kardex form

b. writing "K" in ink in the symbol column in front of the order on the doctor's order sheet to indicate completion of the documentation

5. Recheck each step for accuracy.

6. Sign off the order to indicate completion of transcription.

Place a check mark (✓) in the following box to indicate that you have completed Activity 14-9.

☐ Transcribe a Blood Bank Order   Date: _____

◎ ACTIVITY 14-10

TRANSCRIBE URINALYSIS/URINE CHEMISTRY ORDERS

Materials Needed   Black ink pen

Red ink pen (depending on hospital policy)

Pencil

Eraser

Kardex form used in Activity 14-9

Patient ID labels (if using requisition method)

Laboratory requisition form (if using requisition method)

Computer and Practice Activity Software for Transcription of Physicians' Orders

Directions

Refer to Physicians' Order Sheet 14-10 in your patient's chart. Practice transcribing the urinalysis orders by performing the following steps. Check with your instructor for variations of the procedure to adapt it to the practice in your area. Place a check mark (✓) in the box as you complete each step.

Steps for Transcribing Urinalysis/Urine Chemistry Orders

1. Read the orders. ❏

2. Obtain the Kardex form and a requisition form if using the requisition method. ❏

3. Order the tests from the laboratory department. ❏

Use the computer and practice software by:
  a. selecting Enter Orders on the home screen ❏
  b. selecting the patient's name from the census on the viewing screen ❏
  c. selecting the laboratory department from the department menu on the viewing screen ❏
  d. selecting the urinalysis division from the laboratory department viewing screen ❏
  e. typing in the pertinent information ❏
  f. selecting the tests to be ordered from the menu on the viewing screen ❏
  g. writing "ord" in ink above each order on the doctor's order sheet to indicate that the test has been ordered ❏
  h. when collected, checking the label on the specimen for proper patient ID, date, and time collected, and for the initials of the person who collected the specimen ❏
  i. sending the specimen with a copy of the order to the laboratory ❏

> ★ **HIGH PRIORITY**
>
> Usually the order is entered into the computer when the specimen is obtained. Attach a copy of the order from the computer. Because this specimen is obtained by an invasive procedure, it cannot be sent by a tube system. It must be hand-carried to the laboratory.

Use the requisition form by:
  a. affixing the patient's ID label to the form ❏

> ★ **HIGH PRIORITY**
>
> Each urine specimen may require a separate requisition and label because the specimens may go to different divisions of the laboratory. For example, urine osmolality would be done in the chemistry department and urine culture and sensitivity would be done in the microbiology department.

  b. writing in the pertinent information on the requisition form ❏
  c. placing a check mark (✓) in the column next to the tests to be ordered ❏
  d. writing "ord" in ink above each order on the doctor's order sheet to indicate that the test has been ordered ❏
  e. when collected, checking the label on the specimen for proper patient ID, date, and time collected, and for the initials of the person who collected the specimen ❏
  f. sending the specimen with a copy of the order to the laboratory ❏

4. Document the orders by:
  a. writing the date and the order in pencil in the laboratory column on the Kardex form ❏
  b. writing "K" in ink in the symbol column in front of the order on the doctor's order sheet to indicate completion of the documentation ❏

5. Recheck each step for accuracy. ❏

6. Sign off the orders to indicate completion of transcription. ❏

Place a check mark (✓) in the following box to indicate that you have completed Activity 14-10.

☐ Transcribe Urinalysis/Urine Chemistry Orders   Date: _____

◎ ACTIVITY 14-11

TRANSCRIBE CEREBROSPINAL FLUID ORDERS

Materials Needed   Black ink pen

Red ink pen (depending on hospital policy)

Pencil

Eraser

Kardex form used in Activity 14-10

Patient ID labels (if using requisition method)

Laboratory requisition forms (if using requisition method)

Central service department (CSD) requisition (if using requisition method)

Consent form

Computer and Practice Activity Software for Transcription of Physicians' Orders

Directions

Refer to Physicians' Order Sheet 14-11 in your patient's chart. Practice transcribing the cerebrospinal fluid orders by performing the following steps. Check with your instructor for variations of the procedure to adapt it to the practice in your area. Place a check mark (✓) in the box as you complete each step.

Steps for Transcribing Cerebrospinal Fluid Orders

1. Read the orders.   ☐

2. Obtain the Kardex form, a consent form, and a requisition form if using the requisition method.   ☐

★ HIGH PRIORITY

A lumbar puncture is an invasive procedure used to obtain cerebral spinal fluid. A consent form must be prepared and signed by the patient. Refer to Activity 8-5 for the steps to prepare a consent form. The consent order is usually transcribed onto the Kardex form. A lumbar puncture tray will need to be ordered if not in the CSD supply locker.

---

3. Order the tests from the laboratory department.   ☐

★ HIGH PRIORITY

Specimen bottles should be bagged with the patient ID label with the date, time, and the initials of the person who collected the specimen written on the label. Numbers are etched on the specimen bottles. Indicate the tube number next to the name of the test on the requisition. The numbers refer to the first specimen of fluid obtained (1), the second specimen of fluid (2), and the third specimen of fluid (3). The doctor will indicate which test he or she wants on each tube by number.

Use the computer and practice software by:

   a. affixing the patient's ID label to the consent form ☐

   b. writing in the pertinent information on the consent form ☐

   c. giving the consent form to the patient's nurse for the patient to sign ☐

   d. selecting Enter Orders on the home screen ☐

   e. selecting the patient's name from the census on the viewing screen ☐

   f. selecting the laboratory department from the department menu on the viewing screen ☐

   g. selecting the fluids division from the laboratory department viewing screen ☐

   h. typing in the pertinent information ☐

   i. selecting the body cavity source from the menu on the viewing screen ☐

   j. selecting the tests to be ordered from the menu on the viewing screen ☐

   k. writing "ord" in ink above each order on the doctor's order sheet to indicate that the test has been ordered ☐

   l. checking the label on each specimen for proper patient ID, date, and time collected, and for the initials of the person who collected the specimen ☐

   m. sending the specimens with a copy of the order to the laboratory ☐

Use the requisition form by:

   a. affixing the patient's ID labels to the requisition form and the consent form ☐

   b. writing in the pertinent information on the consent form ☐

   c. giving the consent form to the patient's nurse for the patient to sign ☐

   d. writing in the pertinent information on the requisition ☐

   e. placing a check mark (✓) in the column next to the tests to be ordered ☐

   f. writing "ord" in ink above each order on the doctor's order sheet to indicate that the test has been ordered ☐

   g. checking each label for proper patient ID, date, and time collected, and for the initials of the person who collected the specimen ☐

   h. sending the specimens with a copy of the order to the laboratory ☐

4. Document the orders by:

   a. writing the date and order in pencil in the laboratory column on the Kardex form ☐

   b. writing "K" in ink in the symbol column in front of the order on the doctor's order sheet to indicate completion of the documentation ☐

5. Recheck each step for accuracy. ☐

6. Sign off the orders to indicate completion of transcription. ☐

Place a check mark (✓) in the following box to indicate that you have completed Activity 14-11.

☐ Transcribe Cerebrospinal Fluid Orders   Date: _____

⊚ ACTIVITY 14-12

TRANSCRIBE A REVIEW SET OF LABORATORY ORDERS

Materials Needed

Black ink pen

Red ink pen (depending on hospital policy)

Pencil

Eraser

Kardex form used in Activity 14-11

Patient ID labels (if using requisition method)

Laboratory requisition forms (if using requisition method)

Computer and Practice Activity Software for Transcription of Physicians' Orders

Directions

Refer to Physicians' Order Sheet 14-12 in your patient's chart. Transcribe the orders. Refer to previous laboratory activities for the appropriate transcription steps as needed.

Steps for Transcribing a Review Set of Laboratory Orders

1. Read the orders. ❑
2. Check orders for stats. ❑
3. Place and document telephone call for notification of stats. ❑
4. Obtain the Kardex form and requisition forms if using the requisition method. ❑
5. Order as necessary. ❑
6. Document the orders on the Kardex form. ❑
7. Recheck each step for accuracy. ❑
8. Sign off the orders to indicate completion of transcription. ❑

★ HIGH PRIORITY

Transcribing doctors' orders is a critical task, and an error could cause harm to a patient. If you are not absolutely sure when interpreting the doctor's orders, ask the patient's nurse or the doctor who wrote the orders.

Place a check mark (✓) in the following box to indicate that you have completed Activity 14-12.

❑ Transcribe a Review Set of Laboratory Orders   Date: _____

ACTIVITY 14-13

TRANSCRIBE A REVIEW SET OF DOCTORS' ORDERS

Materials Needed

Black ink pen
Red ink pen (depending on hospital policy)
Pencil
Yellow highlighter
Eraser
Kardex form and medical administration record (MAR) used in previous chapters
Patient ID labels (if using requisition method)
Necessary requisition forms

Directions

Refer to Physicians' Order Sheet 14-13 in your patient's chart. Transcribe the orders. Refer to the previous activities for the appropriate transcription steps as needed.

Steps for Transcribing a Review Set of Doctors' Orders

1. Read the complete set of doctors' orders. ❑
2. Send the pharmacy copy. ❑
3. Check orders for stats. ❑
4. Make any necessary phone calls. ❑
5. Obtain all necessary forms. ❑

   6. Order as necessary.   ❑

   7. Document the orders on the Kardex form.   ❑

   8. Document the medications on the MAR.   ❑

   9. Recheck each step for accuracy.   ❑

   10. Sign off the orders to indicate completion of transcription.   ❑

Suggestion to the student: Use this space to list the forms you will need.

Place a check mark (✓) in the following box to indicate that you have completed Activity 14-13.

❑ Transcribe a Review Set of Doctors' Orders   Date: _____

ACTIVITY 14-14

TRANSCRIBE TELEPHONE MESSAGES

Materials Needed   Pen or pencil
                         Note pad

Directions

Practice transcribing the following printed telephone messages by performing the following steps. Place a check mark (✓) in the box as you complete each step.

Telephone Messages

1. "Hi. This is Pat in chemistry. Would you check with Dr. Black to find out if the potassium that she ordered on Johnny Smith this afternoon can be run on the blood we have on him from this morning?"

2. "Hi there! This is Jenny in hemo. Would you let Scott Martin's nurse know that the specimen that was just drawn for the stat potassium was hemolyzed, and we need to get a new specimen?"

3. "This is John in micro. Please let Susan Garcia's nurse know that there is insufficient quantity to do all of the cultures on the stool specimen that she sent us."

Steps for Transcribing Telephone Messages

1. Have someone read these messages to you while you transcribe them on a note pad.   ❑

2. Write down for whom the message is intended.   ❑

3. Write down the caller's name.   ❑

4. Write down the date and time of the call.   ❑

5. Write down the purpose of the call.   ❑

6. If a return call is expected, write down the number to call.   ❑

7. Sign your name to the message.   ❑

Place a check mark (✓) in the following box to indicate that you have completed Activity 14-14.

☐ Transcribe Telephone Messages   Date: _____

ACTIVITY 14-15

TRANSCRIBE TELEPHONED LABORATORY RESULTS

Materials Needed   Pen or pencil
Laboratory result form

Directions

Practice transcribing the following laboratory results by performing the following steps. Place a check mark (✓) in the box as you complete each step.

Telephoned Laboratory Results

1. "Hi, this is Jeannie from chemistry in the lab. I have stat electrolyte results on Terita Banks. Are you ready?
Sodium = 136 mEq/L
Potassium = 3.8 mEq/L
Chloride = 106 mEq/L
CO_2 = 21 mEq/L
Please repeat those back to me. Thanks."

2. "This is Chuck from hematology in the lab. I have some coag results on Frances Key.

PT was 12 seconds
INR was 2
PTT was 24.2 seconds
Repeat those please. Thanks."

3. "This is Jennifer from chemistry in the lab with a critical potassium value on Megan Morgan. The potassium was 7.2. Please repeat the value and ask the resident if she would like a repeat venous specimen drawn and run. May I have your name again please? Thanks."

4. "Hi, this is Joe from chemistry in the lab. I have stat cardiac labs on Pat Tagler. Ready?
CPK = 250 mU/mL
LDH = 200 mU/mL
AST = 45 IU/L
BNP = 90 pg/mL
Troponin I = 0.025 ng/mL
Would you repeat those results please? Thanks."

Steps for Transcribing Telephoned Laboratory Results

1. Have someone read these laboratory results to you while you write them on a laboratory result form.   ☐

2. Repeat the results back to the person giving them to you.   ☐

3. Write the name of the person giving you the results.   ☐

4. Notify the patient's nurse of the results and, if necessary (requested by the nurse or previously requested by resident or doctor), the patient's resident or doctor.   ☐

Place a check mark (✓) in the following box to indicate that you have completed Activity 14-15.

☐ Transcribe Telephone Laboratory Results   Date: _____

PHYSICIANS' ORDER SHEET 14-1

DATE	TIME	SYMBOL	ORDERS
03/12	0700	K, ORP	CBC
		K, ORP	LE cell prep ⎫ today
		K, ORP	Retic count ⎬
			Dr.
			Mar 12/20, 0710, C. DeSantis, HUC

PHYSICIANS' ORDER SHEET 14-2

DATE	TIME	SYMBOL	ORDERS
03/13	0700	K, ORP	Daily H & H ⎫ starting
		K, ORP	PT/INR qd ⎬ in am
			Dr.
			Mar 13/20, 0710 C. Desantis, HUC

PHYSICIANS' ORDER SHEET 14-3

DATE	TIME	SYMBOL	ORDERS
03/14	0700	K, ORD	lytes
		K, ORD	Mg ⎫ this am
		K, ORD	uric acid ⎬
			Dr.
			Mar 14/20, 0710 C. DeSantis, HUC

PHYSICIANS' ORDER SHEET 14-4

DATE	TIME	SYMBOL	ORDERS
03/15	0700	K, ORD	Stat CK-MB, Troponin & BNP
		K, ORD	RBS now
			Dr.
			Mar 15/20, 0710, C. De Santis, HUC

PHYSICIANS' ORDER SHEET 14-5

DATE	TIME	SYMBOL	ORDERS
03/16	0700		FBS
			chol
			trig in am
			Fe, TIBC & ferritin (tomorrow)
			Dr.
			Mar 16/20, 0705, C. De Santis, HUC.

PHYSICIANS' ORDER SHEET 14-6

DATE	TIME	SYMBOL	ORDERS
03/17	0700	K	D/C daily H&H
		K, ORD	Stat BMP
		K, ORD	2 hr PP BS today
		K, ORD	serum osmolality today
		K, ORD	Daily FBS
		K, ORD	Thyroid Profile in am
		K, ORD	Vancomycin peak & trough around 6pm dose
			Dr.
			Mar 17/20, 0710 C. De Santis, HUC.

PHYSICIANS' ORDER SHEET 14-7

DATE	TIME	SYMBOL	ORDERS
			Reflex UA
			Sputum for AFB culture and C&S
			Blood C&S x 2 sites
			Stool x 3 for O & P
			Dr.

PHYSICIANS' ORDER SHEET 14-8

DATE	TIME	SYMBOL	ORDERS
			RA factor
			EBV panel
			ANA profile
			CMV IgG & IgM by Elisa
			Anti-VZV by PCR
			Serum immunoelectrophoresis
			Dr.

PHYSICIANS' ORDER SHEET 14-9

DATE	TIME	SYMBOL	ORDERS
			T & X-match 2 u PC for transfusion today
			Dr.

PHYSICIANS' ORDER SHEET 14-10

DATE	TIME	SYMBOL	ORDERS
			Rout UA
			Urine osmolality
			Dr.

PHYSICIANS' ORDER SHEET 14-11

DATE	TIME	SYMBOL	ORDERS
			Have consent signed for LP per Dr. Sarah Bellum
			CSF to lab for:
			Tube #1—cell ct c̄ diff
			Tube #2—protein & gluc
			Tube #3—C & S & anaerobic Cx
			Tube #4—HSV IgM and CMV IgM by PCR
			Dr.

PHYSICIANS' ORDER SHEET 14-12

DATE	TIME	SYMBOL	ORDERS
			H&H, K and Na today q 1-2h per ISTAT until c̄ in normal limits;
			other studies done in lab
			ESR & creatinine
			Bilirubin total & indirect } today
			Cocci screen—to Dr. Pappagianis' lab
			CK-MB & troponin now and in 8 hrs
			CMP & HgA1C in am
			Dr.

PHYSICIANS' ORDER SHEET 14-13

DATE	TIME	SYMBOL	ORDERS
			D/C fluid restrictions
			encourage ambulation
			obtain ETS
			reinsert Foley—strict I & O
			Start IVF of 1000 mL Ionosol T @ 100mL/hr
			D/C temazepam
			Sliding Scale as follows; Humalog
			200 — 250 — 5 units
			251 — 300 — 10 units
			301 — 350 — 15 units
			NPH Insulin 10 units sq q HS
			cath urine for UA & C & S
			Coag profile
			BMP, CBC, Mg, & ionized Ca q am
			Dr.

CHAPTER 15

Diagnostic Imaging Orders

Activities in this Chapter:

★ HIGH PRIORITY

When the electronic medical record (EMR) with computerized physician order entry system has been implemented, the doctor will enter orders directly into the patient's EMR. The orders will automatically be sent to the diagnostic imaging department. The health unit coordinator (HUC) may communicate with the diagnostic imaging department regarding scheduling of the procedures. The HUC may also order food trays when a patient returns to the room after completing a procedure for which they were fasting. The paper-based requisition methods are included for learning purposes.

★ HIGH PRIORITY

Review Chapter 15 in *LaFleur Brooks' Health Unit Coordinating,* 7th edition, for explanations of doctors' orders, diagnostic imaging procedures, and definitions of abbreviations.

Place the Physicians' Order Sheets located at the end of the chapter in your patient's chart. Follow the directions for each activity to transcribe orders.

ACTIVITY 15-1

TRANSCRIBE RADIOLOGY (X-RAY) ORDERS THAT DO NOT REQUIRE PREPARATION OR CONTRAST MEDIUM

Materials Needed   Black ink pen

Red ink pen (depending on hospital policy)

Pencil

Eraser

Kardex form used in previous chapters

Patient ID labels (if using requisition method)

Diagnostic imaging requisition form (if using requisition method)

Computer and Practice Activity Software for Transcription of Physicians' Orders

Directions

Refer to Physicians' Order Sheet 15-1 in your patient's chart. Practice transcribing the radiology orders by performing the following steps. Check with your instructor for variations of the procedure to adapt it to the practice in your area. Place a check mark (✓) in the box as you complete each step.

Steps for Transcribing Radiology (X-ray) Orders That Do Not Require Preparation or Contrast Medium

1. Read the orders. ❑

2. Obtain the Kardex form and requisition form if using the requisition method. ❑

3. Order the studies from the diagnostic imaging department. ❑

Use the computer and the practice software by:

  a. selecting Enter Orders on the home screen ❑

  b. selecting the patient's name from the census on the viewing screen ❑

  c. selecting the diagnostic imaging department from the department menu on the viewing screen ❑

  d. selecting the appropriate division from the diagnostic imaging divisions screen ❑

  e. typing in the pertinent data and answering all questions asked on computer screen (i.e., reason for examination, transportation method, whether patient is on oxygen, whether patient has an intravenous [IV] line) ❑

  f. entering the study(s) to be performed ❑

  g. entering the date each study is to be performed under the appropriate heading ❑

  h. writing "ord" in ink above each order on the doctor's order sheet to indicate that the study has been ordered ❑

  i. sending the order by pressing Enter Order(s) on the viewing screen ❑

Use the requisition form by:

  a. affixing the patient's ID label to the form ❑

  b. writing in the pertinent information and answering all questions asked on requisition (i.e., reason for examination, transportation method, whether patient is on oxygen, whether patient has an IV line) ❑

  c. writing the order under the heading Examination Requested ❑

  d. writing the date each study is to be performed in the appropriate space ❑

  e. writing "ord" in ink above each order on the doctor's order sheet to indicate that the study has been ordered ❑

  f. sending the requisition ❑

4. Document the orders by:

  a. writing the date and order in pencil in the diagnostic imaging column on the Kardex form ❑

  b. writing in pencil the date the radiology study will be performed in the column next to the order ❑

  c. writing "K" in ink in the symbol column in front of the order on the doctor's order sheet to indicate completion of the documentation ❑

5. Recheck each step for accuracy. ❑

6. Sign off the orders to indicate completion of transcription. ❑

Place a check mark (✓) in the following box to indicate that you have completed Activity 15-1.

☐ Transcribe Radiology (X-ray) Orders That Do Not
Require Preparation or Contrast Medium   Date: _____

ACTIVITY 15-2

TRANSCRIBE RADIOLOGY ORDERS THAT REQUIRE PREPARATION AND CONTRAST MEDIUM

Materials Needed   Black ink pen
Red ink pen (depending on hospital policy)
Pencil
Eraser
Kardex form used in Activity 15-1
Labeled medication administration record (MAR) used in previous chapters
Patient ID labels (if using requisition method)
Nutritional care requisition form (if using requisition method)
Diagnostic requisition forms (if using requisition method)
Diagnostic imaging routine preparation directions (printed at the end of this chapter)
Computer and Practice Activity Software for Transcription of Physicians' Orders

Directions

Refer to Physicians' Order Sheet 15-2 in your patient's chart. Practice transcribing the radiology orders by performing the following steps. Check with your instructor for variations of the procedure in your area. Place a check mark (✓) in the box as you complete each step.

Steps for Transcribing Radiology Orders That Require Preparation and Contrast Medium

1. Read the orders.   ☐

2. Obtain the Kardex form, diagnostic imaging routine preparation directions, MAR, and requisition   ☐
forms if using the requisition method.

★ HIGH PRIORITY

Many health care facility computer systems automatically provide a printout of the appropriate diagnostic imaging preparation directions when the examination is ordered.

3. Order the studies from the diagnostic imaging department.   ☐
Use the computer and practice software by:
a. selecting Enter Orders on the home screen   ☐
b. selecting the patient's name from the census on the viewing screen   ☐
c. selecting the diagnostic imaging department from the department menu on the viewing
screen   ☐
d. selecting the appropriate division from the diagnostic imaging divisions screen   ☐
e. typing in the pertinent data and answering all questions asked on the computer screen
(i.e., reason for examination, transportation method, whether patient is on oxygen, whether
patient has an IV line)   ☐

  f. entering each study to be performed ❑
  g. entering the date each study is to be performed under the appropriate heading ❑
  h. writing "ord" in ink above each order on the doctor's order sheet to indicate that the study has been ordered ❑
  i. sending the order by pressing Enter Order(s) on the viewing screen ❑
  j. placing the diagnostic imaging preparation printout with the patient's Kardex form ❑

Use the requisition form by:
  a. affixing the patient's ID label to the form ❑
  b. writing in the pertinent information and answering all questions asked on requisition (i.e., reason for examination, transportation method, whether patient is on oxygen, whether patient has an IV line)
  c. writing the order under the heading Examination Requested ❑
  d. writing the date each study is to be performed in the appropriate space ❑
  e. writing "ord" in ink above each order on the doctor's order sheet to indicate that the study has been ordered ❑
  f. sending the requisition ❑
  g. placing the diagnostic imaging preparation card with the patient's Kardex form ❑

4. Order the diet change from the nutritional care department by entering the diet change into the computer or by using the diet requisition form (refer to the nutritional care activities in Chapter 12 in this manual). ❑

★ **HIGH PRIORITY**

The diet change order in the routine preparation may need to be documented on the original physician's orders. This may be done by writing "diet ord" or "prep ord" to the right of the orders in red ink.

---

5. Document the orders by:
  a. writing the date and order in pencil in the diagnostic imaging column on the Kardex form ❑
  b. writing in pencil the date the radiology study will be performed in the column next to the order ❑
  c. writing "K" in ink in the symbol column in front of the order on the doctor's order sheet to indicate completion of the documentation ❑

★ **HIGH PRIORITY**

The preparation directions computer printout or preparation direction card is often placed with the patient's Kardex form in the file; therefore the preparation and diet for the procedure usually does not need to be written on the Kardex form.

---

6. Document the preparation medication (obtained from the preparation directions) in ink on the MAR under the correct heading by:
  a. writing (1) today's date, (2) the name of the medication, (3) the dosage, (4) the route of administration, (5) the time of administration, and (6) the date of administration ❑
  b. writing "m" in ink in the symbol column in front of the order on the doctor's order sheet to indicate completion of the documentation ❑

7. Recheck each step for accuracy. ❑
8. Sign off the orders to indicate completion of transcription. ❑

Place a check mark (✓) in the following box to indicate that you have completed Activity 15-2.

❑ Transcribe Radiology Orders That Require Preparation and Contrast Medium

Date: _____

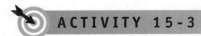

ACTIVITY 15-3

TRANSCRIBE A SPECIAL RADIOLOGY PROCEDURE ORDER

Materials Needed

Black ink pen

Red ink pen (depending on hospital policy)

Pencil

Eraser

Kardex form used in Activity 15-2

Labeled MAR used in Activity 15-2

Patient ID labels

Nutritional care requisition form (if using requisition method)

Diagnostic imaging requisition form (if using requisition method)

Consent form for operation, administration of anesthetics, and the rendering of other medical services form

Computer and Practice Activity Software for Transcription of Physicians' Orders

Directions

Refer to Physicians' Order Sheet 15-3 in your patient's chart. Practice transcribing the special radiology procedure order and related orders by performing the following steps. Check with your instructor for variations of the procedure to adapt it to the practice in your area. Place a check mark (✓) in the box as you complete each step.

Steps for Transcribing a Special Radiology Procedure Order

1. Read the order.

2. Obtain the Kardex form, MAR, consent form, and requisition form if using the requisition method.

3. Order the procedure from the diagnostic imaging department.

Use the computer and practice software by:

    a. affixing the patient's ID label and writing in the procedure on the consent form

    b. filling in the procedure on the consent form and giving it to the patient's nurse for the patient to sign

    c. selecting Enter Orders on the home screen

    d. selecting the patient's name from the census on the viewing screen

    e. selecting the diagnostic imaging department from the department menu on the viewing screen

    f. selecting the appropriate division from the diagnostic imaging divisions screen

    g. typing in the pertinent data and answering all questions asked on the computer screen (i.e., reason for examination, transportation method, whether patient is on oxygen, whether patient has an IV line)

    h. entering the procedure to be performed

    i. entering the date the procedure is to be performed under the appropriate heading

    j. writing "ord" in ink above each order on the doctor's order sheet to indicate that the procedure has been ordered

    k. sending the order by pressing Enter Order(s) on the viewing screen

Use the requisition form by:

    a. affixing the patient's ID label and writing in the procedure on the consent form

    b. filling in the procedure on the consent form and giving it to the patient's nurse for the patient to sign

    c. affixing the patient's ID label to the diagnostic imaging requisition form

    d. writing in the pertinent information and answering all questions asked on the requisition (i.e., reason for examination, transportation method, whether patient is on oxygen, whether patient has an IV line)

    e. writing the order under the heading Examination Requested

    f. writing the date the procedure is to be performed in the appropriate space

    g. writing "ord" in ink above each order on the doctor's order sheet to indicate that the procedure has been ordered   ☐

    h. sending the requisition   ☐

4. Order the diet change from the nutritional care department by using the computer or the requisition form (refer to the nutritional care activities in Chapter 12 in this manual).   ☐

> **⭐ HIGH PRIORITY**
>
> The patient is usually restricted to nothing by mouth (NPO) for special procedures.

5. Document the radiology order by:

    a. writing the date and order in pencil in the diagnostic imaging column on the Kardex form   ☐

    b. writing in pencil the date the radiology procedure will be done in the column next to the order   ☐

    c. writing "K" in ink in the symbol column in front of the order on the doctor's order sheet to indicate completion of the documentation   ☐

6. Document the diet change by:

    a. writing the date and order in pencil in the diet column on the Kardex form   ☐

    b. writing "K" in ink in the symbol column in front of the order on the doctor's order sheet to indicate completion of the documentation   ☐

7. Document the medications in ink on the MAR under the correct heading by:

    a. writing (1) today's date, (2) the name of the medication, (3) the dosage, (4) the route of administration, (5) the time of administration, and (6) the date of administration   ☐

    b. writing "m" in ink in the symbol column in front of the order on the doctor's order sheet to indicate completion of the documentation   ☐

8. Recheck each step for accuracy.   ☐

9. Sign off the orders to indicate completion of transcription.   ☐

Place a check mark (✓) in the following box to indicate that you have completed Activity 15-3.

☐ Transcribe a Special Radiology Procedure Order   Date: _____

◎ ACTIVITY 15-4

TRANSCRIBE A COMPUTED TOMOGRAPHY ORDER, AN ULTRASOUND ORDER, AND A MAGNETIC RESONANCE IMAGING ORDER

Materials Needed
    Black ink pen
    Red ink pen (depending on hospital policy)
    Pencil
    Eraser
    Kardex form used in Activity 15-3
    Patient ID labels
    Diagnostic imaging requisition form (if using the requisition method)
    Computer and Practice Activity Software for Transcription of Physicians' Orders

Directions

Refer to Physicians' Order Sheet 15-4 in your patient's chart. Practice transcribing the diagnostic imaging orders by performing the following steps. Check with your instructor for variations of the procedure to adapt it to the practice in your area. Place a check mark (✓) in the box as you complete each step.

Steps for Transcribing a Computed Tomography Order, an Ultrasound Order, and a Magnetic Resonance Imaging Order

1. Read the orders. ☐

2. Obtain the Kardex form and requisition forms if using the requisition method. ☐

3. Order each study from the diagnostic imaging department. ☐

Use the computer and practice software by:

   a. selecting Enter Orders on the home screen ☐

   b. selecting the patient's name from the census on the viewing screen ☐

   c. selecting the diagnostic imaging department from the department menu on the viewing screen ☐

   d. selecting the appropriate division from the diagnostic imaging divisions screen ☐

   e. typing in the pertinent data and answering all questions on the computer screen (i.e., reason for examination, transportation method, whether patient is on oxygen, whether patient has an IV line) ☐

   f. entering each study to be performed ☐

   g. entering the date each study is to be performed under the appropriate heading ☐

   h. writing "ord" in ink above each order on the doctor's order sheet to indicate that the study has been ordered ☐

   i. sending the order by pressing Enter Order(s) on the viewing screen ☐

Use the requisition form by:

   a. affixing the patient's ID label to the form ☐

   b. writing in the pertinent information and answering all questions asked on the requisition (i.e., reason for examination, transportation method, whether patient is on oxygen, whether patient has an IV line) ☐

   c. writing the order under the heading Examination Requested ☐

   d. writing the date the study is to be performed in the appropriate space ☐

   e. writing "ord" in ink above each order on the doctor's order sheet to indicate that the study has been ordered ☐

> ⭐ **HIGH PRIORITY**
>
> The patient may be kept NPO for some computed tomography (CT), ultrasound (US), or magnetic resonance imaging procedures. Check with your instructor for directions.

4. If necessary, order the diet change from the nutritional care department by using the computer or the requisition form (refer to the nutritional care activities in Chapter 12 in this manual). ☐

> ⭐ **HIGH PRIORITY**
>
> Diagnostic imaging studies usually need to be entered separately into the computer, or separate requisitions are usually used if the studies are to be performed by different divisions in the diagnostic imaging department.

5. Document the orders by:

   a. writing the date and order in pencil in the diagnostic imaging column on the Kardex form ☐

   b. writing in pencil the date the radiology study will be performed in the column next to the order ☐

   c. writing "K" in ink in the symbol column in front of the order on the doctor's order sheet to indicate completion of the documentation ☐

6. Recheck each step for accuracy. ☐

7. Sign off the orders to indicate completion of transcription. ☐

Place a check mark (✓) in the following box to indicate that you have completed Activity 15-4.

☐ Transcribe a Computed Tomography Order, an Ultrasound Order, and a Magnetic Resonance Imaging Order   Date: _____

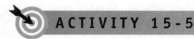

ACTIVITY 15-5

TRANSCRIBE A NUCLEAR MEDICINE ORDER

Materials Needed   Black ink pen

Red ink pen (depending on hospital policy)

Pencil

Eraser

Kardex form used in Activity 15-4

Patient ID labels (if using requisition method)

Diagnostic imaging requisition form (if using requisition method)

Computer and Practice Activity Software for Transcription of Physicians' Orders

Directions

Refer to Physicians' Order Sheet 15-5 in your patient's chart. Practice transcribing the nuclear medicine order by performing the following steps. Check with your instructor for variations of the procedure to adapt it to the practice in your area. Place a check mark (✓) in the box as you complete each step.

Steps for Transcribing a Nuclear Medicine Order

1. Read the order. ❑

2. Obtain the Kardex form. ❑

3. Order the study from the diagnostic imaging department. ❑

Use the computer and practice software by:

  a. selecting Enter Orders on the home screen ❑

  b. selecting the patient's name from the census on the viewing screen ❑

  c. selecting the diagnostic imaging department from the department menu on the viewing screen ❑

  d. selecting the nuclear medicine division from the viewing screen ❑

  e. typing in the pertinent data and answering all questions on the requisition (i.e., reason for examination, transportation method, whether patient is on oxygen, whether patient has an IV line) ❑

  f. entering the study to be performed ❑

  g. entering the date the study is to be performed under the appropriate heading ❑

  h. writing "ord" in ink above each order on the doctor's order sheet to indicate that the study has been ordered ❑

  i. sending the order by pressing Enter Order(s) on the viewing screen ❑

Use the requisition form by:

  a. affixing the patient's ID label to the form ❑

  b. writing in the pertinent information and answering all questions on the requisition (i.e., reason for examination, transportation method, whether patient is on oxygen, whether patient has an IV line) ❑

  c. writing the order under the heading Examination Requested ❑

  d. writing the date the study is to be performed in the appropriate space ❑

  e. writing "ord" in ink above each order on the doctor's order sheet to indicate that the study has been ordered ❑

  f. sending the requisition ❑

4. Document the orders by:

  a. writing the date and order in pencil in the diagnostic imaging column on the Kardex form ❑

  b. writing in pencil the date the radiology study will be performed in the column next to the order ❑

  c. writing "K" in ink in the symbol column in front of the order on the doctor's order sheet to indicate completion of the documentation ❑

5. Recheck each step for accuracy. ❑

6. Sign off the orders to indicate completion of transcription. ❑

Place a check mark (✓) in the following box to indicate that you have completed Activity 15-5.

❏ Transcribe a Nuclear Medicine Order   Date: _____

ACTIVITY 15-6

TRANSCRIBE A REVIEW SET OF DOCTORS' ORDERS

Materials Needed   Black ink pen
                         Red ink pen (depending on hospital policy)
                         Pencil
                         Eraser
                         Yellow highlighter
                         Kardex form used in Activity 15-5
                         Patient ID labels
                         Necessary requisition forms
                         Computer and Practice Activity Software for Transcription of Physicians' Orders

Directions

Refer to Physicians' Order Sheet 15-6 in your patient's chart. Transcribe the orders. Refer to the previous activities for the appropriate transcription steps as needed.

Steps for Transcribing a Review Set of Doctors' Orders

1. Read the orders.   ❏
2. Send or fax the pharmacy copy.   ❏
3. Check orders for stats.   ❏
4. Make any necessary phone calls.   ❏
5. Obtain all necessary forms and radiology preparation cards.   ❏
6. Order as necessary.   ❏
7. Document the order on the Kardex form.   ❏
8. Document medications on the MAR.   ❏
9. Recheck each step for accuracy.   ❏
10. Sign off the orders to indicate completion of transcription.   ❏

> Suggestion to the student: Use this space to list the forms you will need.

Place a check mark (✓) in the following box to indicate that you have completed Activity 15-6.

❏ Transcribe a Review Set of Doctors' Orders   Date: _____

ACTIVITY 15-7

TRANSCRIBE RECORDED TELEPHONE MESSAGES

Materials Needed   Pen or pencil

Note pad

Directions

Practice transcribing the following printed telephone messages by performing the following steps. Place a check mark (✓) in the box as you complete each step.

Telephone Messages

1. "This is Paul in radiology. We are ready for John Fracture to do his chest X-ray examination. Please notify his nurse that someone will be up in 5 minutes to pick him up."

2. "Hi, this is Cindy in CT. Could you have Pat Simon's nurse arrange to have him down for a CT of the brain at 1:00 PM sharp? If there is a problem please call me right back. Thanks."

3. "This is Paula in special procedures. Please ask Mary Copa's nurse to give the on-call med ordered and we will be up to get her in half an hour. Thanks."

Steps for Transcribing Recorded Telephone Messages

1. Have someone read the above messages to you while you write them on a note pad. ❑

2. Write down for whom the message is intended. ❑

3. Write down the caller's name. ❑

4. Write down the date and time of the call. ❑

5. Write down the purpose of the call. ❑

6. If a return call is expected, write down the number to call. ❑

7. Sign your name to the message. ❑

Place a check mark (✓) in the following box to indicate that you have completed Activity 15-7.

❑ Transcribe Recorded Telephone Messages   Date: _____

DIAGNOSTIC IMAGING ROUTINE PREPARATION DIRECTIONS

Directions

Cut appropriate preparation direction along dotted line. Document medications (including packaged enemas) on your patient's MAR. Place the prep card with your patient's Kardex form.

Note: Preparations for diagnostic procedures vary among hospitals. (Check with your instructor for any variations in these directions.)

IVU OR IVP

Cleansing tap H_2O enema the evening prior to procedure

Ensure adequate hydration (IV or oral) before and after the procedure to prevent dye-induced renal failure

NPO 8-12 hours before procedure

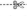

UGI-SBFT

NPO 8-12 hours before procedure

No smoking or gum chewing 8-12 hours before procedure

BE

Day before procedure:

Clear liquids (no dairy products) for lunch and dinner

Magnesium of citrate 1 bottle @ 1400

Bisacodyl 5 mg 2 tabs @ 1900

NPO 2400 hrs

Tap H_2O enema @ 0600 day of procedure

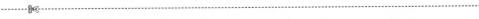

US OF ABDOMEN

NPO 8-12 hours before procedure

Full bladder, drink H_2O—Do not void

No smoking AM prior to procedure

US OF PELVIS

Full bladder, drink H_2O—Do not void

No H_2O is needed if US is to be done vaginally only

US OF GB

Fat-free PM meal day before procedure

Fast 8-10 hours prior to procedure

No smoking AM prior to procedure

PHYSICIANS' ORDER SHEET 15-1

DATE	TIME	SYMBOL	ORDERS
03/	0700	K, ORD	PA & lat chest Cl: ✓ for infiltrates
		K, ORD	KUB Cl: acute abd
			Dr.
			J. Ruiz March 30/19 7:10 HUC
		K, ORD	Mammogram Cl: tumor
			Dr.
			J. Ruiz, March 30/19, 7

PHYSICIANS' ORDER SHEET 15-2

DATE	TIME	SYMBOL	ORDERS
03/31	0700	K, ORD	IVU Cl: poss ureterolithiasis
		K, ORD.	BE Cl: ✓ for polyps
			Dr.
			Mar 31/20, 0710, C. De Santis, HUC.

PHYSICIANS' ORDER SHEET 15-3

DATE	TIME	SYMBOL	ORDERS
04/01	0700	K, ORD	Venogram lt leg Cl: Severe edema
			have consent signed
PC		M, ORD	Demerol 100 mg ⎤ IM
sent		M, ORD	Vistaril 25 mg ⎦ 0730
		M, ORD	NPO 2400
			Dr.
			April 1/ 20, 0710, C. De Santis, HUC.

PHYSICIANS' ORDER SHEET 15-4

DATE	TIME	SYMBOL	ORDERS
			CT of chest c̄ and s̄ contrast CI: poss aneurysm
			US of abd CI: abscess
			MRI of lt shoulder CI: torn rotator cuff
			Dr.

PHYSICIANS' ORDER SHEET 15-5

DATE	TIME	SYMBOL	ORDERS
			VQ study stat CI: poss PE
			Dr.

PHYSICIANS' ORDER SHEET 15-6

DATE	TIME	SYMBOL	ORDERS
			Δ diet to mech soft 1500 cal ADA
			VS q4hr—call hospitalist if diastolic ≥ 90 or if C/O SOB
			Repeat cath UA & C & S
			Δ IVF to 1000 mls Isolite M @ 120 mls/hr
			p̄ urine obtained, start doxycycline 500 mg IVPB q day
			Tylenol 650 mg po q4h prn fever
			D/C temazepam
			Start Ambien 5 mg PO qhs
			Δ warfarin to 5 mg Mon—Thur & 2.5 mg F, Sat & Sun
			stat PCXR CI: poss infiltrates
			UGI c̄ SBFT CI: peptic ulcer
			lymphangiogram lt leg CI: poss lymphatic obst
			stat H & H & repeat in 2 hr
			Δ daily PT/INR to q Mon & Thurs
			T & X 2 units PC to hold
			Dr.

CHAPTER 16

Other Diagnostic Studies

Activities in this Chapter:

★ HIGH PRIORITY

When an electronic medical record (EMR) with computerized physician order entry system has been implemented, the doctor will enter orders directly into the patient's EMR. The orders will automatically be sent to the diagnostic department. The health unit coordinator (HUC) may communicate with the diagnostic department regarding scheduling of the procedures. The HUC may also order food trays when patients return to their rooms after completing a procedure for which they were fasting. The paper-based requisition methods are included for learning purposes.

★ HIGH PRIORITY

Review Chapter 16 in *LaFleur Brooks' Health Unit Coordinating*, 7th edition, for explanations of doctors' orders, diagnostic tests, and definitions of abbreviations.

Place the Physicians' Order Sheets located at the end of the chapter in your patient's chart. Follow the directions for each activity to transcribe orders.

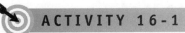

ACTIVITY 16-1

TRANSCRIBE NEUROLOGY ORDERS

Materials Needed
Black ink pen
Red ink pen (depending on hospital policy)
Pencil
Eraser
Kardex form used in previous chapter
Medication administration record (MAR) used in previous chapters
Patient ID labels (if using the requisition method)
Neurology department requisition form (if using the requisition method)
Computer and Practice Activity Software for Transcription of Physicians' Orders

Directions

Refer to Physicians' Order Sheet 16-1 in your patient's chart. Practice transcribing the neurology order by performing the following steps. Check with your instructor for variations of the procedure to adapt it to the practice in your area. Place a check mark (✓) in the box as you complete each step.

Steps for Transcribing Neurology Orders

1. Read the order. ❑

2. Obtain the Kardex form and requisition form if using the requisition method. ❑

3. Order the study from the neurology department. ❑

Use the computer and the practice software by:
a. selecting Enter Orders on the home screen ❑
b. selecting the patient's name from the census on the viewing screen ❑
c. selecting the neurology department from the department menu on the viewing screen ❑
d. typing in the pertinent data (refer to your patient's MAR)—enter any anticonvulsive medications your patient is taking on the computer screen ❑
e. entering the study to be performed ❑

> ### ⭐ HIGH PRIORITY
>
> It is important for the neurologist who is interpreting the results of the study to know if the patient is taking an anticonvulsive medication or a medication for sedation. Refer to Chapter 13 in *LaFleur Brooks' Health Unit Coordinating*, 7th edition, for a list of these medications. Enter any anticonvulsive medications into the computer or write them on the requisition.

---

f. writing "ord" in ink above each order on the doctor's order sheet to indicate that the study has been ordered ❑
g. sending the order by pressing Enter Order(s) on the viewing screen ❑

Use the requisition form by:
a. affixing the patient's ID label to the form ❑
b. writing in the pertinent information (refer to your patient's MAR)—write any anticonvulsive medications that your patient is taking on the requisition ❑
c. placing a check mark (✓) in the box next to the study to be ordered ❑
d. writing "ord" in ink above each order on the doctor's order sheet to indicate that the study has been ordered ❑
e. sending the requisition ❑

4. Document the order by:
   a. writing the date and order in pencil in the diagnostic studies column on the Kardex form
   b. writing in pencil the date that the neurology order will be done in the column next to the order
   c. writing "K" in ink in the symbol column in front of the order on the doctor's order sheet to indicate completion of the documentation

5. Recheck each step for accuracy.

6. Sign off the orders to indicate completion of transcription.

Place a check mark (✓) in the following box to indicate that you have completed Activity 16-1.

☐ Transcribe Neurology Orders   Date: _____

⊙ ACTIVITY 16-2

TRANSCRIBE CARDIOVASCULAR DIAGNOSTIC ORDERS

Materials Needed   Black ink pen

Red ink pen (depending on hospital policy)

Pencil

Eraser

Kardex form used in Activity 16-1

MAR used in Activity 16-1

Patient ID labels (if using the requisition method)

Cardiovascular diagnostics requisition form (if using the requisition method)

Computer and Practice Activity Software for Transcription of Physicians' Orders

Directions

Refer to Physicians' Order Sheet 16-2 in your patient's chart. Practice transcribing the cardiovascular diagnostic orders by performing the following steps. Check with your instructor for variations of the procedure to adapt it to the practice in your area. Place a check mark (✓) in the box as you complete each step.

Steps for Transcribing Cardiovascular Diagnostics Orders

1. Read the orders.

2. Obtain the Kardex form and requisition form if using the requisition method.

3. Order the studies from the cardiovascular diagnostics department. It is important for the cardiologist interpreting the results of the studies to know if the patient is taking cardiovascular medications. Refer to Chapter 13 in *LaFleur Brooks' Health Unit Coordinating,* 7th edition, for a list of cardiovascular medications. Document those that have been ordered for the patient on the requisition or enter the medications into the computer.

Use the computer and the practice software by:
   a. selecting Enter Orders on the home screen
   b. selecting the patient's name from the census on the viewing screen
   c. selecting the cardiovascular department from the department menu on the viewing screen
   d. typing in the pertinent information (refer to your patient's MAR)—enter any cardiovascular medications onto the order screen
   e. entering the study to be performed
   f. entering the date the study is to be performed under the appropriate heading

> ⭐ **HIGH PRIORITY**
>
> When filling out the requisition for a cardiovascular test, the HUC may need to identify whether the patient is currently on cardiovascular medication. This information is entered in the computer or written on the requisition. Studies ordered on different days usually require separate orders. Most health care facility computer systems can order tests for future dates.

   g. writing "ord" in ink above each order on the doctor's order sheet to indicate that the study has been ordered ☐

   h. sending the order by pressing Enter Order(s) on the viewing screen ☐

Use the requisition form by:

   a. affixing the patient's ID label to the form ☐

   b. writing in the pertinent information (refer to your patient's MAR)—write any cardiovascular medications that your patient is taking on the requisition ☐

   c. placing a check mark (✓) in the box next to the study to be ordered ☐

   d. writing the date and the study to be performed in the appropriate space ☐

   e. writing "ord" in ink above each order on the doctor's order sheet to indicate that the study has been ordered ☐

   f. sending the requisition ☐

4. Document the orders by:

   a. writing the date and order in pencil in the diagnostic studies column on the Kardex form ☐

   b. writing in pencil the date that the cardiovascular study will be done in the column next to the order ☐

   c. writing "K" in ink in the symbol column in front of the order on the doctor's order sheet to indicate completion of the documentation ☐

5. Recheck each step for accuracy. ☐

6. Sign off the orders to indicate completion of transcription. ☐

Place a check mark (✓) in the following box to indicate that you have completed Activity 16-2.

☐ Transcribe Cardiovascular Diagnostic Orders   Date: _____

⌖ ACTIVITY 16-3

TRANSCRIBE ENDOSCOPY ORDERS

Materials Needed   Black ink pen

Red ink pen (depending on hospital policy)

Pencil

Eraser

Kardex form used in Activity 16-2

Patient ID labels

Consent form for procedure

Diet requisition form

Computer and Practice Activity Software for Transcription of Physicians' Orders

Telephone

Directions

Refer to Physicians' Order Sheet 16-3 on your patient's chart. Practice transcribing the endoscopy order and the related orders by performing the following steps. Check with your instructor for variations of the procedure to adapt it to the practice in your area. Place a check mark (✓) in the box as you complete each step.

Steps for Transcribing an Endoscopy Order

1. Read the orders. ❑

2. Obtain the Kardex form, diet requisition form, and consent to procedure form. ❑

> ⭐ **HIGH PRIORITY**
>
> An endoscopy is usually scheduled by the doctor performing the examination. The date and time of the procedure may be included in the doctor's orders. The endoscopy department should be called to verify the schedule. Some hospitals may require the order to be entered into the computer for billing purposes. A consent form is required for an endoscopy procedure. Refer to Activity 8-5 for the steps to prepare a consent form.

3. Schedule the endoscopy examination (or verify if scheduled by doctor) by:
   a. calling the endoscopy department to determine the date and time of the procedure ❑

> ⭐ **HIGH PRIORITY**
>
> Notify the endoscopy department of the patient's name, unit, room number, and diagnosis. The department will inform you of the time the examination is scheduled. Document the information on the Kardex form. A call to the doctor's office to notify the doctor of the time of examination may be necessary.

   b. preparing the consent form and writing "prepared" above the endoscopy order on the order sheet ❑

4. Enter the order into the computer or send a requisition for billing purposes. ❑

5. Order the diet change from the nutritional care department by computer or by using the requisition form. (Refer to the nutritional care activities in Chapter 12 in this manual.) ❑

6. Document the order by:
   a. writing the date and order in pencil in the diagnostic studies column on the Kardex form ❑
   b. writing the scheduled date and time in pencil in the column next to the order ❑
   c. writing "K" in ink in the symbol column in front of the order on the doctor's order sheet to indicate completion of the documentation ❑

7. Document the nothing-by-mouth order by:
   a. writing the date and order in the diet column on the Kardex form ❑
   b. writing "K" in ink in the symbol column in front of the order on the doctor's order sheet to indicate completion of the documentation ❑

8. Recheck each step for accuracy. ❑

9. Sign off the orders to indicate completion of transcription. ❑

Place a check mark (✓) in the following box to indicate that you have completed Activity 16-3.

❑ Transcribe Endoscopy Orders   Date: _____

ACTIVITY 16-4

TRANSCRIBE CARDIOPULMONARY (RESPIRATORY CARE) DIAGNOSTIC ORDERS

Materials Needed
Black ink pen
Red ink pen (depending on hospital policy)
Pencil
Eraser
Kardex form used in Activity 16-3
MAR used in previous chapters
Patient ID labels (if using the requisition method)
Cardiopulmonary (respiratory care) diagnostics requisition form (if using the requisition method)
Computer and Practice Activity Software for Transcription of Physicians' Orders

Directions

Refer to Physicians' Order Sheet 16-4 in your patient's chart. Practice transcribing the cardiopulmonary (respiratory care) diagnostics order by performing the following steps. Check with your instructor for variations of the procedure to adapt it to the practice in your area. Place a check mark (✓) in the box as you complete each step.

Steps for Transcribing Cardiopulmonary (Respiratory Care) Diagnostics Orders

1. Read the order. ❑
2. Obtain the Kardex form and requisition form if using the requisition method. ❑
3. Order the study from the cardiopulmonary (respiratory care) department. ❑

Use the computer and the practice software by:
  a. selecting Enter Orders on the home screen ❑
  b. selecting the patient's name from the census on the viewing screen ❑
  c. selecting the cardiopulmonary department from the department menu on the viewing screen ❑
  d. selecting the diagnostics division from the viewing screen ❑
  e. typing in the pertinent information (refer to your patient's MAR)—enter any anticoagulant medications that your patient is taking onto the order screen ❑
  f. entering the study to be performed ❑
  g. writing "ord" in ink above each order on the doctor's order sheet to indicate that the study has been ordered ❑
  h. sending the order by pressing Enter Order(s) on the viewing screen ❑

Use the requisition form by:
  a. affixing the patient's ID label to the cardiopulmonary (respiratory care) form ❑
  b. writing in the pertinent information (refer to your patient's MAR)—write any anticoagulant medications that your patient is taking on the requisition ❑
  c. placing a check mark (✓) in the box next to the cardiopulmonary (respiratory care) order ❑
  d. writing "ord" in ink above each order on the doctor's order sheet to indicate that the study has been ordered ❑

★ HIGH PRIORITY

When filling out the requisition for an arterial blood gas study, the HUC may need to identify whether the patient is currently on anticoagulant medication. This information is entered in the computer or written on the requisition.

  e. sending the requisition ❑

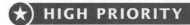

★ HIGH PRIORITY

The cardiopulmonary (respiratory care) department performs both diagnostic tests and treatments. Many hospital units now use point-of-care testing to obtain arterial blood gas levels, in which case the nursing staff collects and tests the specimen.

4. Document the order by:
   a. writing the date and order in pencil in the pulmonary function column on the Kardex form ☐
   b. writing "K" in ink in the symbol column in front of the order on the doctor's order sheet to indicate completion of the documentation ☐
5. Recheck each step for accuracy. ☐
6. Sign off the order to indicate completion of transcription. ☐

Place a check mark (✓) in the following box to indicate that you have completed Activity 16-4.

☐ Transcribe Cardiopulmonary (Respiratory Care) Diagnostics Orders

Date: _____

◎ ACTIVITY 16-5

TRANSCRIBE A REVIEW SET OF DOCTORS' ORDERS

Materials Needed   Black ink pen

Red ink pen (depending on hospital policy)

Pencil

Eraser

Kardex form used in Activity 16-4

MAR used in Activity 16-4

Patient ID labels

All necessary forms and requisitions

Computer and Practice Activity Software for Transcription of Physicians' Orders

Directions

Refer to Physicians' Order Sheet 16-5 in your patient's chart. Transcribe the orders. Refer to previous activities for the appropriate steps as needed.

Steps for Transcribing a Review Set of Doctors' Orders

1. Read the orders. ☐
2. Send or fax the pharmacy copy. ☐
3. Check orders for stats. ☐
4. Make any necessary telephone calls. ☐
5. Obtain all necessary forms and requisitions. ☐

> Suggestion to the student: Use this space to list the forms you will need.

6. Order as necessary. ☐
7. Prepare consent forms as required. ☐
8. Document the orders on the Kardex form. ☐
9. Document the medications on the MAR. ☐
10. Recheck each step for accuracy. ☐
11. Sign off the orders to indicate completion of transcription. ☐

⭐ **HIGH PRIORITY**

Transcribing doctors' orders is a critical task, and an error could cause harm to a patient. If you are not absolutely sure when interpreting the doctor's orders, ask the patient's nurse or the doctor who wrote the orders.

Place a check mark (✓) in the following box to indicate that you have completed Activity 16-5.

☐ Transcribe a Review Set of Doctors' Orders   Date: _____

🎯 **ACTIVITY 16-6**

TRANSCRIBE RECORDED TELEPHONE MESSAGES

Materials Needed   Pen or pencil
                              Note pad

Directions

Practice transcribing the following printed telephone messages by performing the following steps. Place a check mark (✓) in the box as you complete each step.

Telephone Messages

1. "Hi, this is Jane in the cath lab. Would you check with Mary Copa's nurse to make sure that Mary has stopped taking anticoags? Thanks."

2. "Hi, this is Pete in endoscopy. Please ask John Smith's nurse to give the on-call medication now. We will be up to get him in 20 minutes; please have his chart ready. Thanks."

Steps for Transcribing Recorded Telephone Messages

1. Have someone read these messages to you while you write them on a note pad. ❑

2. Write down for whom the message is intended. ❑

3. Write down the caller's name. ❑

4. Write down the date and time of the call. ❑

5. Write down the purpose of the call. ❑

6. If a return call is expected, write down the number to call. ❑

7. Sign your name to the message. ❑

Place a check mark (✓) in the following box to indicate that you have completed Activity 16-6.

❑ Transcribe Recorded Telephone Messages   Date: _____

PHYSICIANS' ORDER SHEET 16-1

DATE	TIME	SYMBOL	ORDERS
			EEG to eval sz activity
			EMG of lower extremities in a.m. to assess muscle weakness
			AEP to eval hearing loss
			page Dr. Sarah Bellum c̄ results of EEG
			Dr.

PHYSICIANS' ORDER SHEET 16-2

DATE	TIME	SYMBOL	ORDERS
			EKG c̄ rhythm strip now
			2 D M-mode echo
			Carotid Doppler today
			Dr.

PHYSICIANS' ORDER SHEET 16-3

DATE	TIME	SYMBOL	ORDERS
			EGD @ 0800 tomorrow
			NPO @ MN
			Consent per Dr. Colin Packer
			Dr.

PHYSICIANS' ORDER SHEET 16-4

DATE	TIME	SYMBOL	ORDERS
			PFTs c̄ & s̄ bronchodilator
			ABG on RA—page me c̄ results
			Con't pulse ox
			Dr.

PHYSICIANS' ORDER SHEET 16-5

DATE	TIME	SYMBOL	ORDERS
			1500 cal ADA low-chol diet
			amb c̄ help bid — to 100 ft in hallway as tol
			TEE today
			Repeat ABG now
			PA & lat chest films CI: cocci vs pertussis
			CK-MB & troponin I now and q8h X 2 sets
			CRP & CMP stat
			CMP, Mg & phos in a.m.
			sputum for AFB cx & stain
			convert IV to HL c̄ rout saline flushes
			Head CT s̄ contrast in AM CI: poss tumor
			Call Dr. Phoebe Martin for consult re chest pain
			Dr.
			Consent for cardiac cath for EP studies in a.m. per Dr. P. Martin
			lorazepam 10 mg IM on call to cath lab
			NPO 2400 hrs
			DC warfarin, Plavix and ASA
			May have small sips to take a.m. meds
			Dr.

CHAPTER 17

Treatment Orders

Activities in this Chapter:

★ HIGH PRIORITY

When the electronic medical record (EMR) with computerized physician order entry system has been implemented, the doctor will enter orders directly into the patient's EMR. The orders will automatically be sent to the appropriate departments. The health unit coordinator (HUC) may communicate with the various departments regarding scheduling of the procedures. The paper-based requisition methods are included for learning purposes.

★ HIGH PRIORITY

Review Chapter 17 in *LaFleur Brooks' Health Unit Coordinating,* 7th edition, for explanations of doctors' orders and definitions of abbreviations.

Place the Physicians' Order Sheets located at the end of the chapter in your patient's chart. Follow the directions for each activity to transcribe orders.

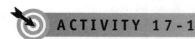

ACTIVITY 17-1

TRANSCRIBE CARDIOVASCULAR THERAPY (TREATMENT) ORDERS

Materials Needed

Black ink pen

Red ink pen (depending on hospital policy)

Pencil

Eraser

Kardex form used in previous chapters

Medication administration record (MAR) used in previous chapters

Patient ID labels (if using the requisition method)

Cardiovascular diagnostics requisition form (if using the requisition method)

Consent form

Computer and Practice Activity Software for Transcription of Physicians' Orders

Directions

Refer to Physicians' Order Sheet 17-1 in your patient's chart. Practice transcribing the cardiovascular therapy (treatment) orders by performing the following steps. Check with your instructor for variations of the procedure to adapt it to the practice in your area. Place a check mark (✓) in the box as you complete each step.

Steps for Transcribing Cardiovascular Therapy (Treatment) Orders

1. Read the orders. ☐

2. Obtain the Kardex form, consent form, and requisition form if using the requisition method. ☐

3. Order the studies from the cardiovascular diagnostics department. It is important for the cardiologist interpreting the results of the studies to know if the patient is taking cardiovascular medications. Refer to Chapter 13 in *LaFleur Brooks' Health Unit Coordinating*, 7th edition, for a list of cardiovascular medications. Document those that have been ordered for the patient on the requisition or enter the medications into the computer. ☐

Use the computer and the practice software by:

  a. affixing the patient's ID label and writing in the procedure on the consent form ☐

  b. filling in the procedure on the consent form and giving it to the patient's nurse for the patient to sign ☐

  c. selecting Enter Orders on the home screen ☐

  d. selecting the patient's name from the census on the viewing screen ☐

  e. selecting the cardiovascular department from the department menu on the viewing screen. The interventional therapy may be listed under "invasive studies." ☐

  f. typing in the pertinent information (refer to your patient's MAR)—enter any cardiovascular medications onto the order screen ☐

  g. entering the treatment to be performed ☐

  h. entering the date the treatment is to be performed under the appropriate heading ☐

★ HIGH PRIORITY

When filling out the requisition for a cardiovascular treatment, the HUC may need to identify whether the patient is currently on cardiovascular medication. If it is an invasive procedure, the HUC may also need to identify whether the patient is on anticoagulant medication (including aspirin). This information is entered in the computer or written on the requisition. Studies ordered on different days usually require separate orders. Most health care facility computer systems can order tests for future dates.

---

  i. writing "ord" in ink above each order on the doctor's order sheet to indicate that the study has been ordered ☐

  j. sending the order by pressing Enter Order(s) on the viewing screen ☐

Use the requisition form by:
   a. affixing the patient's ID label to the form ☐
   b. writing in the pertinent information (refer to your patient's MAR)—write ☐
      any cardiovascular medications that your patient is taking on the requisition
   c. placing a check mark (✓) in the box next to the study to be ordered ☐
   d. writing the date and the study to be performed in the appropriate space ☐
   e. writing "ord" in ink above each order on the doctor's order sheet to ☐
      indicate that the study has been ordered
   f. sending the requisition ☐

4. Document the orders by:
   a. writing the date and order in pencil in the diagnostic studies column on the Kardex form ☐
   b. writing in pencil the date that the cardiovascular treatment will be done in the column next ☐
      to the order
   c. writing "K" in ink in the symbol column in front of the order on the ☐
      doctor's order sheet to indicate completion of the documentation
5. Recheck each step for accuracy. ☐
6. Sign off the orders to indicate completion of transcription. ☐

Place a check mark (✓) in the following box to indicate that you have completed Activity 17-1.

☐ Transcribe Cardiovascular Therapy (Treatment) Orders   Date: _____

◎ ACTIVITY 17-2

TRANSCRIBE CARDIOPULMONARY (RESPIRATORY CARE) TREATMENT ORDERS

Materials Needed   Black ink pen
                     Red ink pen (depending on hospital policy)
                     Pencil
                     Eraser
                     Kardex form used in Activity 17-1
                     Patient ID labels (if using requisition method)
                     Cardiopulmonary (respiratory care) requisition form (if using requisition method)
                     Computer and Practice Activity Software for Transcription of Physicians' Orders

Directions

Refer to Physicians' Order Sheet 17-2 in your patient's chart. Practice transcribing the cardiopulmonary (respiratory care) treatment orders by performing the following steps. Check with your instructor for variations of the procedure to adapt it to the practice in your area. Place a check mark (✓) in the box as you complete each step.

Steps for Transcribing Cardiopulmonary (Respiratory Care) Treatment Orders

1. Read the orders. ☐
2. Obtain the Kardex form and cardiopulmonary (respiratory care) department requisition form if ☐
   using the requisition method.
3. Order the cardiopulmonary (respiratory) care treatments and equipment from the ☐
   cardiopulmonary (respiratory care) department.
Use the computer and the practice software by:
   a. selecting Enter Orders on the home screen ☐
   b. selecting the patient's name from the census on the viewing screen ☐
   c. selecting the cardiopulmonary department from the department menu on the viewing screen ☐

d. selecting the appropriate division from the cardiopulmonary (respiratory care) divisions screen ☐
e. typing in the pertinent information ☐
f. selecting treatments and equipment to be ordered from the menu on the screen ☐
g. writing "ord" in ink above each order on the doctor's order sheet to indicate that the treatments and equipment have been ordered ☐
h. sending the order by pressing Enter Order(s) on the viewing screen ☐

Use the requisition form by:
a. affixing the patient's ID label to the form ☐
b. writing in the pertinent information ☐
c. placing a check mark (✓) in the box next to the cardiopulmonary (respiratory care) treatments and equipment to be ordered (writing any special instructions in the space provided) ☐
d. writing "ord" in ink above each order on the doctor's order sheet to indicate that the cardiopulmonary (respiratory care) treatments or equipment have been ordered ☐
e. sending the requisition ☐

⭐ **HIGH PRIORITY**

Albuterol (Ventolin), ipratropium (Atrovent), pirbuterol (Maxair), budesonide (Pulmicort), beclomethasone (Vanceril), fluticasone (Flovent), triamcinolone (Azmacort), acetylcysteine (Mucomyst), gentamicin, and tobramycin are some of the medications commonly used with cardiopulmonary (respiratory care) treatments. It is important that the HUC write the entire doctor's order (including medications) when sending a treatment order to the cardiopulmonary (respiratory care) department.

---

4. Document the orders by:
a. writing the date and order in pencil in the cardiopulmonary (respiratory care) column on the Kardex form ☐
b. writing "K" in ink in the symbol column in front of the order on the doctor's order sheet to indicate completion of the documentation ☐

5. Recheck each step for accuracy. ☐

6. Sign off the orders to indicate completion of transcription. To transcribe a doctor's order to discontinue cardiopulmonary (respiratory care), enter the discontinued order into the computer. It may be necessary to notify the cardiopulmonary (respiratory care) department by telephone. Write "called" and the time called next to the order on the doctor's order sheet to indicate completion of the call. ☐

Place a check mark (✓) in the following box to indicate that you have completed Activity 17-2.

☐ Transcribe Cardiopulmonary (Respiratory Care)
Treatment Orders

Date: _____

🎯 **ACTIVITY 17-3**

TRANSCRIBE TRACTION ORDERS

Materials Needed   Black ink pen

Red ink pen (depending on hospital policy)

Pencil

Eraser

Kardex form used in Activity 17-2

Patient ID labels (if using requisition method)

Central service department (CSD) requisition form (if using requisition method)

Computer and Practice Activity Software for Transcription of Physicians' Orders

Directions

Refer to Physicians' Order Sheet 17-3 in your patient's chart. Practice transcribing the traction orders by performing the following steps. Check with your instructor for variations of the procedure to adapt it to the practice in your area. Place a check mark (✓) in the box as you complete each step.

Steps for Transcribing Traction Orders

1. Read the orders. ☐

2. Obtain the Kardex form and requisition form if using the requisition method. ☐

3. Order the orthopedic equipment from the CSD. ☐

Use the computer and the practice software by:
- a. selecting Enter Orders on the home screen ☐
- b. selecting the patient's name from the census on the viewing screen ☐
- c. selecting the orthopedic equipment department from the department menu on the viewing screen ☐
- d. typing in the pertinent information ☐
- e. selecting the orthopedic equipment to be ordered from the menu on the viewing screen ☐
- f. writing "ord" in ink in front of the order on the doctor's order sheet to indicate that the orthopedic equipment has been ordered ☐
- g. sending the order by pressing Enter Order(s) on the viewing screen ☐

Use the requisition form by:
- a. affixing the patient's ID label to the form ☐
- b. writing in the pertinent information ☐
- c. placing a check mark (✓) in the box next to the equipment to be ordered ☐
- d. writing "ord" in ink above each order on the doctor's order sheet to indicate that the orthopedic equipment has been ordered ☐
- e. sending the requisition ☐

3. Notify the patient's nurse verbally of the order and document the name of the nurse with the time notified above the order on the doctor's order sheet. ☐

4. Document the orders by:
- a. writing the date and order in pencil in the treatment column on the Kardex form ☐
- b. writing "K" in ink in the symbol column in front of the order on the doctor's order sheet to indicate completion of the documentation ☐

5. Recheck each step for accuracy. ☐

6. Sign off the orders to indicate completion of transcription. ☐

★ HIGH PRIORITY

To transcribe a doctor's order to discontinue traction, notify the patient's nurse and the orthopedic technician (if applicable). Write "notified" or "called" and the time next to the order on the doctor's order sheet to indicate completion of the call. When using a computer, enter the discontinued order into the computer.

Place a check mark (✓) in the following box to indicate that you have completed Activity 17-3.

☐ Transcribe Traction Orders   Date: _____

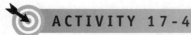

ACTIVITY 17-4

TRANSCRIBE PHYSICAL MEDICINE AND REHABILITATION ORDERS

Materials Needed   Black ink pen

Red ink pen (depending on hospital policy)

Pencil

Eraser

Kardex form used in Activity 17-3

Patient ID labels (if using requisition method)

Physical medicine and rehabilitation requisition forms (if using requisition method)

Computer and Practice Activity Software for Transcription of Physicians' Orders

Directions

Refer to Physicians' Order Sheet 17-4 in your patient's chart. Practice transcribing the physical medicine and rehabilitation orders by performing the following steps. Check with your instructor for variations of the procedure to adapt it to the practice in your area. Place a check mark (✓) in the box as you complete each step.

Steps for Transcribing Physical Medicine and Rehabilitation Orders

1. Read the orders. ❑

2. Obtain the Kardex form and requisition forms if using the requisition method. ❑

3. Order the physical medicine or rehabilitation treatments from the physical medicine and rehabilitation department. ❑

Use the computer and the practice software by:

a. selecting Enter Orders on the home screen ❑

b. selecting the patient's name from the census on the viewing screen ❑

c. selecting the physical medicine department from the department menu on the viewing screen ❑

d. selecting the appropriate division in the physical medicine department ❑

e. typing in the pertinent information ❑

f. entering the complete order ❑

g. writing "ord" above each order on the doctor's order sheet to indicate that the physical medicine or rehabilitation treatment has been ordered ❑

h. sending the order by pressing Enter Order(s) on the viewing screen ❑

Use the requisition form by:

a. affixing the patient's ID label to the form ❑

b. writing in the pertinent information ❑

c. writing the complete orders in the appropriate space on the requisition form ❑

d. writing "ord" in ink above each order on the doctor's order sheet to indicate that the physical medicine or rehabilitation treatments have been ordered ❑

e. sending the requisition ❑

4. Document the orders by:

a. writing the date and order in pencil in the physical medicine column on the Kardex form ❑

b. writing "K" in ink in the symbol column in front of the order on the doctor's order sheet to indicate completion of the documentation ❑

5. Recheck each step for accuracy. ❑

6. Sign off the orders to indicate completion of transcription. ❑

★ HIGH PRIORITY

To transcribe a doctor's order to discontinue physical medicine or rehabilitation treatments, the HUC needs to communicate the order to that department by entering the discontinued order into the computer.

Place a check mark (✓) in the following box to indicate that you have completed Activity 17-4.

☐ Transcribe Physical Medicine and Rehabilitation Orders   Date: _____

◎ **ACTIVITY 17-5**

TRANSCRIBE A REVIEW SET OF DOCTORS' ORDERS

Materials Needed   Black ink pen
                              Red ink pen (depending on hospital policy)
                              Pencil
                              Eraser
                              Kardex form used in Activity 17-4
                              MAR used in previous chapters
                              Patient ID labels (if using requisition method)
                              All necessary forms
                              Computer and Practice Activity Software for Transcription of Physicians' Orders

Directions

Refer to Physicians' Order Sheet 17-5 in your patient's chart. Transcribe the orders. Refer to previous activities for the appropriate steps as needed.

Steps for Transcribing a Review Set of Doctors' Orders

1. Read the orders.   ☐
2. Send or fax the pharmacy copy.   ☐
3. Check orders for stats.   ☐
4. Place any necessary phone calls.   ☐
5. Obtain all necessary forms.   ☐

Suggestion to the student: Use this space to list the forms you will need.

6. Order as necessary.   ☐
7. Document the orders on the Kardex form.   ☐
8. Document the medications on the MAR.   ☐
9. Recheck each step for accuracy.   ☐
10. Sign off the orders to indicate completion of transcription. ☐

> **★ HIGH PRIORITY**
>
> Transcribing doctors' orders is a critical task, and an error could cause harm to a patient. If you are not absolutely sure when interpreting the doctor's orders, ask the patient's nurse or the doctor who wrote the orders.

Place a check mark (✓) in the following box to indicate that you have completed Activity 17-5.

☐ Transcribe a Review Set of Doctors' Orders   Date: _____

◎ ACTIVITY 17-6

TRANSCRIBE RECORDED TELEPHONE MESSAGES

Materials Needed   Pen or pencil
                         Note pad

Directions

Practice transcribing the following printed telephone messages by performing the following steps. Place a check mark (✓) in the box as you complete each step.

Telephone Messages

1. "Hi, this is Hal in PT. We would like to bring Mary Copa down for her whirlpool at 2:00 PM. Would you check with her nurse to see if that time is okay? Thanks."

2. "Hello, this is June in the recovery room. Please tell John Smith's nurse that John is now in the recovery room. Have gastric suction and oxygen set up in his room. I will call when he is ready to return to the unit. Thanks."

Steps for Transcribing Telephone Messages

1. Have someone read the preceding messages to you while you write them on a note pad.   ☐
2. Write down for whom the message is intended.   ☐
3. Write down the caller's name.   ☐
4. Write down the date and time of the call.   ☐
5. Write down the purpose of the call.   ☐
6. If a return call is expected, write down the number to call.   ☐
7. Sign your name to the message.   ☐

Place a check mark (✓) in the following box to indicate that you have completed Activity 17-6.

☐ Transcribe Recorded Telephone Messages   Date: _____

PHYSICIANS' ORDER SHEET 17-1

DATE	TIME	SYMBOL	ORDERS
			Consent for cardiac cath; poss angioplasty; poss PTCA
			c̄ stent placement @ 0730 tomorrow per Dr. P. Martin
			NPO @ MN
			Dr.

PHYSICIANS' ORDER SHEET 17-2

DATE	TIME	SYMBOL	ORDERS
			40% O_2, 4 L/min NP—titrate to SaO2 $\geq$ 90
			SVN c̄ 0.5 mL albuterol in 2 mL NS q4h c̄ CPT
			induced sputum for C & S, anaerobic and fungal Cxs
			Dr.

PHYSICIANS' ORDER SHEET 17-3

DATE	TIME	SYMBOL	ORDERS
			Bucks tx 10# to lt leg
			OH frame & trapeze
			Dr.

PHYSICIANS' ORDER SHEET 17-4

DATE	TIME	SYMBOL	ORDERS
			DC bucks tx
			PT for crutch training WBAT lt leg
			US & ES to lt leg bid
			PT for ROM lt leg bid
			OT for eval & tx
			Dr.

PHYSICIANS' ORDER SHEET 17-5

DATE	TIME	SYMBOL	ORDERS
			1200 cal ADA diet—FF
			Pedal pulses c̄ VS q 8 hr
			Orthostatic BP qid
			If symptomatic hypotension–lower HOB to flat as tol
			Stat ECG—LOC, then prn chest pain
			Echo today—R/O thrombus
			MUGA scan CI: cardiomyopathy
			MRA of mesenteric vessels CI: poss abscess
			D/C Cipro
			Tobramycin 500 mg IVPB qd
			fluconazole 400 mg PO today, then 200 mg PO qd
			Insert PICC & start IVF of 1000 mL 0.45 NS c̄ 40 mEq
			KCL @ 120 mL/hr
			Daily wt @0700
			D/C foley & send cath for C&S, anaerobic & fungal cx
			Dr.
			EEG
			Stat lytes—call me c̄ results
			Tobramycin level in am
			IS X 10 qhr W/A and prn
			D/C O$_2$
			Δ ROM lt leg to qd
			Δ SVN to q 6 hr
			Consult Dr. Bob Hart re: EF of 25%
			Dr.

Miscellaneous Orders

Activities in this Chapter:

★ HIGH PRIORITY

When the electronic medical record (EMR) with computerized physician order entry system has been implemented, the doctor will enter orders directly into the patient's EMR. The orders will automatically be sent to the appropriate departments. The health unit coordinator (HUC) may communicate with the various departments regarding scheduling of procedures and other issues. The HUC will monitor the patient's EMRs for HUC tasks that will be indicated by an icon (usually a telephone).

★ HIGH PRIORITY

Review Chapter 18 in *LaFleur Brooks' Health Unit Coordinating,* 7th edition, for explanations of doctors' miscellaneous orders and definitions of abbreviations.

Place the Physicians' Order Sheets located at the end of the chapter in your patient's chart. Follow the directions for each activity to transcribe orders.

ACTIVITY 18-1

TRANSCRIBE A CONSULTATION ORDER

Materials Needed	Black ink pen
	Red ink pen (depending on hospital policy)
	Pencil
	Eraser
	Telephone
	Simulated doctors' roster provided in the Practice Activity Software for Transcription of Physicians' Orders
	Kardex form used in previous chapters

Situation

You are working as a health unit coordinator on 5W, a cardiovascular unit, at Opportunity Medical Center. A patient's doctor writes a consultation order for a patient.

Directions

Refer to Physicians' Order Sheet 18-1 in your patient's chart. Practice transcribing the consultation order using the previous situation. Perform the following steps. Check with your instructor for variations of the procedure to adapt it to the practice in your area. Place a check mark (✓) in the box as you complete each step.

Steps for Transcribing a Consultation Order

1. Read the order. ☐

2. Write the following information on your note pad. ☐

NOTE PAD

Consulting doctor's name and telephone number: _____

_____

Hospital name: _____

Patient's name: _____

Patient's location (unit and room number): _____

Name of the doctor requesting the consultation: _____

Patient's diagnosis: _____

---

3. Communicate the order by:
  a. finding the doctor's information in the simulated doctor's roster provided in the Practice Activity Software for Transcription of Physicians' Orders (if using the computer with software) and telephoning the doctor's office or answering service using the information in step 2 ☐
  b. writing "called" and the name or operator number of the person you spoke to, the time you called, and your initials in ink above the order or in the right margin of the doctor's order sheet to indicate the doctor's office has been notified ☐

4. Obtain the Kardex form and simulated doctor's roster. ☐

5. Document the order by:
   a. writing the date and order in pencil in the consultation column on the Kardex form ❑
   b. writing "K" in ink in the symbol column in front of the order on the doctor's order sheet to indicate completion of the documentation ❑

6. Recheck each step for accuracy. ❑

7. Sign off the order to indicate completion of transcription. ❑

★ HIGH PRIORITY

In some hospital units, physicians are required or may wish to call the consulting physician themselves so that the patient's history and other information may be given.

Place a check mark (✓) in the following box to indicate that you have completed Activity 18-1.

❑ Transcribe a Consultation Order　　　　　　Date: _____

ACTIVITY 18-2

TRANSCRIBE A HEALTH INFORMATION MANAGEMENT ORDER

Materials Needed　　Black ink pen
　　　　　　　　　　　　Red ink pen (depending on hospital policy)
　　　　　　　　　　　　Pencil
　　　　　　　　　　　　Eraser
　　　　　　　　　　　　Kardex form used in Activity 18-1
　　　　　　　　　　　　Telephone

Directions

Refer to Physicians' Order Sheet 18-2 in your patient's chart. Practice transcribing the order for obtaining the health records by performing the following steps. Check with your instructor for variations of the procedure to adapt it to the practice in your area. Place a check mark (✓) in the box as you complete each step.

Steps for Transcribing a Health Information Management Order

1. Read the order. ❑

2. Communicate the order by:
   a. telephoning the health information management department to request that the records of the patient be sent to your unit ❑
   b. writing "called" and the name of the person you spoke to, the time you called, and your initials in ink above the order or in the right margin of the doctor's order sheet to indicate that the health records have been requested ❑

3. Document the order by:
   a. placing a check mark (✓) and the date next to Health Records or writing the information on the Kardex form ❑
   b. writing "K" in ink in the symbol column in front of the order on the doctor's order sheet to indicate completion of the documentation ❑

4. Recheck each step for accuracy. ❑

5. Sign off the order to indicate completion of transcription. ❑

★ HIGH PRIORITY

In the hospital setting, the doctor may request records from the patient's previous stay in another hospital. Because the information is confidential, a consent form must be signed by the patient. The consent form will be faxed or scanned and sent electronically to the health information management department of the other hospital. The records will then be released and faxed or sent electronically to the nursing unit.

Place a check mark (✓) in the following box to indicate that you have completed Activity 18-2.

☐ Transcribe a Health Information Management Order   Date: _____

◎ ACTIVITY 18-3

TRANSCRIBE AN ORDER FOR CASE MANAGEMENT

Materials Needed   Black ink pen
Red ink pen (depending on hospital policy)
Pencil
Eraser
Note pad
Kardex form used in Activity 18-2
Telephone
Computer and Practice Activity Software for Transcription of Physicians' Orders

Directions

Refer to Physicians' Order Sheet 18-3 in your patient's chart. Practice transcribing the order for case management by performing the following steps. Check with your instructor for variations of the procedure to adapt it to the practice in your area. Place a check mark (✓) in the box as you complete each step.

Steps for Transcribing an Order for Case Management

1. Read the order.   ☐

2. Communicate the order by:
   a. entering the order into the computer or telephoning the case manager assigned to the patient to relay the doctor's written order   ☐
   b. writing "called," the name of the person you spoke to, the time you called, and your initials in ink above the order or in the right margin of the doctor's order sheet to indicate that the case manager was notified   ☐

3. Document the order by:
   a. writing the date and the order in the appropriate area on the Kardex form   ☐
   b. writing "K" in ink in the symbol column in front of the order on the doctor's order sheet to indicate completion of the documentation   ☐

4. Recheck each step for accuracy.   ☐

5. Sign off the order to indicate completion of transcription.   ☐

★ HIGH PRIORITY

Case managers may work out of the social service department, or they may have a dedicated office in the hospital. Some patients are not assigned a case manager, and a social worker provides support services to the patient and family.

Place a check mark (✓) in the following box to indicate that you have completed Activity 18-3.

❑ Transcribe an Order for Case Management   Date: _____

ACTIVITY 18-4

TRANSCRIBE AN ORDER TO SCHEDULE AN EXAMINATION

Materials Needed   Black ink pen
Red ink pen (depending on hospital policy)
Pencil
Eraser
Note pad
Kardex form used in Activity 18-3
Telephone

Directions

Refer to Physicians' Order Sheet 18-4 in your patient's chart. Practice transcribing the order to schedule an examination by performing the following steps. Check with your instructor for variations of the procedure to adapt it to the practice in your area. Place a check mark (✓) in the box as you complete each step.

Steps for Transcribing an Order to Schedule an Examination

1. Read the order.   ❑

2. Schedule the examination by:
   a. telephoning the appropriate department to arrange an appointment   ❑
   b. writing "called," time of appointment, and the name of the person you spoke to, the time, and your initials in ink above the order or in the right margin of the doctor's order sheet to indicate that the examination has been scheduled   ❑

3. Document the order by:
   a. writing the date and scheduled time and date of the appointment in pencil in the appropriate column on the Kardex form   ❑
   b. writing "K" in ink in the symbol column in front of the order on the doctor's order sheet to indicate completion of the documentation   ❑

4. Recheck each step for accuracy.   ❑

5. Sign off the order to indicate completion of transcription.   ❑

Place a check mark (✓) in the following box to indicate that you have completed Activity 18-4.

❑ Transcribe an Order to Schedule an Examination   Date: _____

ACTIVITY 18-5

TRANSCRIBE A REVIEW SET OF DOCTORS' ORDERS

Materials Needed   Black ink pen
Red ink pen (depending on hospital policy)
Pencil
Eraser

Kardex form used in Activity 18-4

Medication administration record (MAR) used in previous chapters

Telephone

Patient ID labels

All necessary forms

Computer and Practice Activity Software for Transcription of Physicians' Orders

Directions

Refer to Physicians' Order Sheet 18-5 in your patient's chart. Transcribe the orders. Refer to previous activities for the appropriate steps as needed.

Steps for Transcribing a Review Set of Doctors' Orders

1. Read the orders. ❑

2. Send or fax the pharmacy copy. ❑

3. Check orders for stats. ❑

4. Place telephone calls. ❑

5. Obtain all necessary forms. ❑

Suggestion to the student: Use this space to list the forms you will need.

6. Order as necessary. ❑

7. Document the orders on the Kardex form. ❑

8. Document the medications on the MAR. ❑

9. Recheck each step for accuracy. ❑

10. Sign off the orders to indicate completion of transcription. ❑

★ HIGH PRIORITY

Transcribing doctors' orders is a critical task, and an error could cause harm to a patient. If you are not absolutely sure when interpreting the doctor's orders, ask the patient's nurse or the doctor who wrote them.

Place a check mark (✓) in the following box to indicate that you have completed Activity 18-5.

❑ Transcribe a Review Set of Doctors' Orders   Date: _____

★ HIGH PRIORITY

When you have completed Activity 18-5, take all the forms out of your chart. Your patient has been discharged! Your instructor will advise you of the proper procedure in preparing the patient's paper chart for transfer to the health information management department.

PHYSICIANS' ORDER SHEET 18-1

DATE	TIME	SYMBOL	ORDERS
			Dr. Sue Domonas for infectious disease consult ASAP
			Dr.

PHYSICIANS' ORDER SHEET 18-2

DATE	TIME	SYMBOL	ORDERS
			Obtain medical records from previous admissions to this hospital
			Dr.

PHYSICIANS' ORDER SHEET 18-3

DATE	TIME	SYMBOL	ORDERS
			Case Mgt to arrange patient care conference with
			heart transplant team
			Dr.

PHYSICIANS' ORDER SHEET 18-4

DATE	TIME	SYMBOL	ORDERS
			Schedule pt to start radiation tx c̄ Valley Radiology in 1 week
			Dr.

PHYSICIANS' ORDER SHEET 18-5

DATE	TIME	SYMBOL	ORDERS
			Up ad-lib c̄ crutches c̄ assistance
			Chest PA & lat CI: ✓ for infiltrates
			PFTs today
			CBC with manual diff, ESR, CRP, and BMP today—call
			resident c̄ results
			UA this a.m.
			12 lead EKG today—LOC
			Obtain dictated heart cath EP report from HIMS
			Restart O$_2$ at 40% 2L NP
			Con't oximetry
			Call Dr. Rae Chen for poss chemo and biotherapy
			orders
			Dr.
			Social Services to arrange for child care assistance
			Dr.

CHAPTER 19

Admission, Preoperative, and Postoperative Procedures

Activities in this Chapter:

19–1: Admit a Patient to a Nursing Unit
19–2: Transcribe a Set of Admission Orders
19–3: Transcribe a Set of Preoperative Orders
19–4: Transcribe a Set of Postoperative Orders

★ HIGH PRIORITY

When an electronic medical record (EMR) with computerized physician order entry system has been implemented, the doctor will enter orders directly into the patient's EMR. The orders will automatically be sent to the appropriate departments. The health unit coordinator (HUC) may communicate with the various departments regarding scheduling of the procedures. The paper-based requisition methods are included for learning purposes.

★ HIGH PRIORITY

Review admission and preoperative and postoperative procedures in Chapter 19 and locate definitions of abbreviations in Appendix B of *LaFleur Brooks' Health Unit Coordinating,* 7th edition.

Place the Physicians' Order Sheets located at the end of the chapter in your patient's chart. Follow the directions for each activity to transcribe orders.

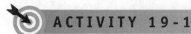

ACTIVITY 19-1

ADMIT A PATIENT TO A NURSING UNIT

Materials Needed

Black ink pen

Red ink pen (depending on hospital policy)

Pencil

Eraser

New Kardex form

New medication administration record (MAR)

Patient ID labels

Standard admission chart forms

Daily census sheet

Admission service agreement form

Computer and Practice Activity Software for Transcription of Physicians' Orders

Face sheet (called patient profile in Practice Activity software)

Situation

A patient is being admitted to the nursing unit at Opportunity Medical Center with a diagnosis of degenerative arthritis. The patient arrives at the unit with an admission service agreement form, a face sheet, and the patient ID labels that have been prepared by the admitting department.

Directions

Place the standard chart forms in your patient's chart. Practice the HUC tasks to admit a patient to the nursing unit using the information in the preceding situation. Ask another student to role-play when necessary in the following steps. Check with your instructor for variations of the procedure to adapt it to the practice in your area. Place a check mark (✓) in the box as you complete each step.

Steps for Admitting a Patient to a Nursing Unit

1. Greet the patient upon arrival at the nurses' station. ❑

> **★ HIGH PRIORITY**
>
> Introduce yourself and give your status. *Example:* "I am (your name), the health unit coordinator for this unit." In some hospitals, the HUC escorts patients to their rooms, instructs them on use of the call button, bed controls, television remote, and internet service (if applicable). The HUC also answers questions regarding visiting hours.

> **★ HIGH PRIORITY**
>
> Add the patient's name to the census using the computer by selecting the admission screen and, if necessary, filling in the pertinent information.

2. Notify the nurse of the patient's arrival and inform the patient that you have notified the nurse. ❑

3. Write the patient's admission on the census sheet and enter the information into the computer if available. ❑

4. Check the patient's signature on the admission service agreement form. ❑

5. If using the computer and Practice Activity Software for Transcription of Physicians' Orders, click on Admission on the home screen and admit a patient (make up a name) using a doctor from the doctors' roster provided in the software. After saving this new patient, click on Patient Profile on the home screen, find this new patient you just admitted, and fill out the patient profile. ❑

> ## ★ HIGH PRIORITY
>
> Compare the spelling of the patient's name on the front sheet and the ID labels. When possible also check the spelling with the patient's signature and on the insurance card. Check to see that the doctor's name is correct.

6. Complete the procedure for the preparation of the chart forms. (Refer to Activity 8-2.) ❑

7. Place the patient ID labels in your patient's chart. ❑

8. Fill in the necessary information on the patient's Kardex form and MAR. ❑

9. Write any allergy information (usually obtained from the nurse's admission notes and doctor's orders) on the front of the patient's chart, the Kardex form, and the MAR. Prepare an allergy bracelet for the patient if necessary. ❑

10. Notify the attending doctor or the hospital resident of the patient's admission. ❑

11. Place the doctor's orders located at the end of this chapter in the patient's chart under the Physicians' Orders tab. ❑

Place a check mark (✓) in the following box to indicate that you have completed Activity 19-1.

❑ Admit a Patient to a Nursing Unit   Date: _____

◎ ACTIVITY 19-2

TRANSCRIBE A SET OF ADMISSION ORDERS

Materials Needed   Black ink pen
Red ink pen (depending on hospital policy)
Pencil
Eraser
Admission order form used in Activity 19-1
Kardex form used in Activity 19-1
MAR used in Activity 19-1
Telephone
Patient ID labels
All necessary forms
Computer and Practice Activity Software for Transcription of Physicians' Orders

Directions

Refer to Physicians' Order Sheet 19-1 in your patient's chart. Transcribe the orders. Refer to previous activities for the appropriate steps as needed.

Steps for Transcribing a Set of Admission Orders

1. Read the orders. ❑

2. Send or fax the pharmacy copy. ❑

3. Check orders for stats. ❑

4. Place telephone calls. ❑
5. Obtain all necessary forms. ❑
6. Order as necessary, using the computer and practice software or requisition forms. ❑
7. Document the orders on the Kardex form. ❑
8. Document the medications on the MAR. ❑
9. Recheck each step for accuracy. ❑
10. Sign off the orders to indicate completion of transcription. ❑

Place a check mark (✓) in the following box to indicate that you have completed Activity 19-2.

❑ Transcribe a Set of Admission Orders   Date: _____

ACTIVITY 19-3

TRANSCRIBE A SET OF PREOPERATIVE ORDERS

Materials Needed   Black ink pen
Red ink pen (depending on hospital policy)
Pencil
Eraser
Kardex form used in Activity 19-2
MAR used in Activity 19-2
Telephone
Patient ID labels
All necessary forms
Computer and Practice Activity Software for Transcription of Physicians' Orders

Directions

Refer to Physicians' Order Sheet 19-2 (from the end of this chapter) in your patient's chart. This order form contains two sets of preoperative orders. Transcribe each set separately. Refer to previous activities for the appropriate steps as needed.

Steps for Transcribing a Set of Preoperative Orders

1. Read the orders. ❑
2. Send or fax the pharmacy copy. ❑
3. Check orders for stats. ❑
4. Place telephone calls. ❑
5. Obtain all necessary forms. ❑
6. Order as necessary, using the computer and practice software or the requisition forms. ❑
7. Document the orders on the Kardex form. ❑
8. Document the medications on the MAR. ❑
9. Recheck all orders for accuracy. ❑
10. Sign off the orders to indicate completion of transcription. ❑

Place a check mark (✓) in the following box to indicate that you have completed Activity 19-3.

❑ Transcribe a Set of Preoperative Orders   Date: _____

ACTIVITY 19-4

TRANSCRIBE A SET OF POSTOPERATIVE ORDERS

Materials Needed   Black ink pen

Red ink pen (depending on hospital policy)

Pencil

Eraser

New Kardex form

New MAR

Telephone

Patient ID labels

All necessary forms

Computer and Practice Activity Software for Transcription of Physicians' Orders

Directions

Refer to Physicians' Order Sheet 19-3 in your patient's chart. Transcribe the orders. Refer to previous activities for the appropriate steps as needed.

Steps for Transcribing a Set of Postoperative Orders

1. Read the orders.   ❑

> **★ HIGH PRIORITY**
>
> All preoperative orders are automatically discontinued postoperatively. The HUC should obtain a new Kardex form and new MAR. The previous MAR should be placed in the patient's chart after the medication divider. Refer to Chapter 19 in *LaFleur Brooks' Health Unit Coordinating*, 7th edition.

2. Send or fax the pharmacy copy.   ❑

3. Check orders for stats.   ❑

4. Place telephone calls.   ❑

5. Obtain all necessary forms.   ❑

6. Order as necessary, using the computer and practice software or the requisition forms.   ❑

7. Document the orders on the Kardex form.   ❑

8. Document the medications on the MAR.   ❑

9. Recheck all orders for accuracy.   ❑

10. Sign off the orders to indicate completion of transcription.   ❑

Place a check mark (✓) in the following box to indicate that you have completed Activity 19-4.

❑ Transcribe a Set of Postoperative Orders   Date: _____

Suggestion to the student: Use this space to list the forms you will need.

PHYSICIANS' ORDER SHEET 19-1

DATE	TIME	SYMBOL	ORDERS
			Admit on observation status to med surg unit
			Dx: Stage III ovarian cancer
			NKDA
			BRP, VS per rout
			Reg diet
			CBC, BMP this a.m., T&C 2 U PC—hold for surg
			UA
			Chest PA & lat —pre-op, EKG—pre-op
			Insert HL c̄ rout saline flushes
			azithromycin 1 g IVPB q12h
			oxycodone 5 mg q4h for pain
			trimethobenzamide 25 mg IM q6h N/V
			zolpidem 30 mg HS for sleep
			Dr.

PHYSICIANS' ORDER SHEET 19-2

DATE	TIME	SYMBOL	ORDERS
			Resp for pre-op teaching
			Foley cath to st. bedside drain
			Start IVF of 1000 mL 0.45 NS @ 120 mL/hr @0600
			Consent for TAH-BSO, expl lap, poss partial colectomy
			Notify Dr. Jane Cohen of pt's admit
			Notify Valley Anesthesia for pre-op orders
			Dr.
			SCDs during surg for DVT prophylaxis
			Abd prep
			NPO 2400
			Demerol 100 mg } *IM*
			Vistaril 25 mg } *0730*
			D/C zolpidem
			temazepam 30 mg PO HS—MR x 1 if nec
			Dr.

PHYSICIANS' ORDER SHEET 19-3

DATE	TIME	SYMBOL	ORDERS
			Admit with IP status
			Rout PACU care
			When stable, trans to SICU
			Primary DX: Stage III ovarian cancer
			S/P TAH, BSO, partial colectomy
			VS & strict I&O q2h X 2, then q4h
			Notify chief resident if: $T > 100 F$, $UOP < 30ml$,
			B/P > 160/100 or < 100/60
			Daily 0700 weight, TCDB q hr WA
			NPO except ice chips, glycerin swabs & hard candy
			IVF: LR @ 125 mL/hr
			Resp for IS q hr WA
			O_2 2 L/M NP
			Morphine Sulfate 2.5 mg IM qh PRN
			Phenergan 25 mg IV push q 6 h PRN
			May D/C Foley when ambulatory
			Apply SCD until ambulatory
			CBC, BMP 0500 & 1600
			ABG 1600—call hospitalist with results
			Dr.
			Mefoxin 1 g IVPB q 8 hr X 3 doses
			Flagyl 500 mg IV Push q8h X 3 doses
			Dr.

CHAPTER 20

Transcribing Discharge Orders

Activities in this Chapter:

20–1: Transcribe an Order for Case Management for Discharge Planning

20–2: Transcribe a Review Set of Doctor's Discharge Orders

★ HIGH PRIORITY

When the electronic medical record (EMR) with computerized physician order entry system has been implemented, the doctor will enter orders directly into the patient's EMR. The orders will automatically be sent to the appropriate departments. The health unit coordinator (HUC) may communicate with the various departments regarding scheduling of procedures and other issues. The HUC will monitor the patient's EMRs for HUC tasks that will be indicated by an icon (usually a telephone).

★ HIGH PRIORITY

Review Chapter 20 in *LaFleur Brooks' Health Unit Coordinating,* 7th edition, for explanations of doctors' miscellaneous orders and definitions of abbreviations.

Place the Physicians' Order Sheets located at the end of the chapter in your patient's chart. Follow the directions for each activity to transcribe orders.

 ACTIVITY 20-1

TRANSCRIBE AN ORDER FOR CASE MANAGEMENT FOR DISCHARGE PLANNING

Materials Needed   Black ink pen

Red ink pen (depending on hospital policy)

Pencil

Eraser

Note pad

Kardex form used in Activity 18-2

Telephone

Computer and Practice Activity Software for Transcription of Physicians' Orders

Directions

Refer to Physicians' Order Sheet 20-1 in your patient's chart. Practice transcribing the order for case management by performing the following steps. Check with your instructor for variations of the procedure to adapt it to the practice in your area. Place a check mark (✓) in the box as you complete each step.

Steps for Transcribing an Order for Case Management for Discharge Planning

1. Read the order. ☐

2. Communicate the order by:
   a. entering the order into the computer or telephoning the case manager assigned to the patient to relay the doctor's written order ☐
   b. writing "called," the name of the person you spoke to, the time you called, and your initials in ink above the order or in the right margin of the doctor's order sheet to indicate that the case manager was notified ☐

3. Document the order by:
   a. writing the date and the order in the appropriate area on the Kardex form ☐
   b. writing "K" in ink in the symbol column in front of the order on the doctor's order sheet to indicate completion of the documentation ☐

4. Recheck each step for accuracy. ☐

5. Sign off the order to indicate completion of transcription. ☐

> ### ★ HIGH PRIORITY
>
> Case managers may work out of the social service department, or they may have a dedicated office in the hospital. Some patients are not assigned a case manager, and a social worker provides support services to the patient and family.

Place a check mark (✓) in the following box to indicate that you have completed Activity 20-1.

☐ Transcribe an Order for Case Management for Discharge Planning   Date: _____

◎ ACTIVITY 20-2

TRANSCRIBE A REVIEW SET OF DOCTOR'S DISCHARGE ORDERS

Materials Needed   Black ink pen

Red ink pen (depending on hospital policy)

Pencil

Eraser

Kardex form used in Activity 18-4

Medication administration record (MAR) used in previous chapters

Telephone

Patient ID labels

All necessary forms

Computer and Practice Activity Software for Transcription of Physicians' Orders

Directions

Refer to Physicians' Order Sheet 20-2 in your patient's chart. Transcribe the orders. Refer to previous activities for the appropriate steps as needed.

Steps for Transcribing a Review Set of Doctors' Discharge Orders

1. Read the orders. ❑
2. Send or fax the pharmacy copy. ❑
3. Check orders for stats. ❑
4. Place telephone calls. ❑
5. Obtain all necessary forms. ❑

Suggestion to the student: Use this space to list the forms you will need.

---

6. Order as necessary. ❑
7. Document the orders on the Kardex form. ❑
8. Document the medications on the MAR. ❑
9. Recheck each step for accuracy. ❑
10. Sign off the orders to indicate completion of transcription. ❑

★ HIGH PRIORITY

Transcribing doctors' orders is a critical task, and an error could cause harm to a patient. If you are not absolutely sure when interpreting the doctor's orders, ask the patient's nurse or the doctor who wrote them.

Place a check mark (✓) in the following box to indicate that you have completed Activity 20-2.

❑ Transcribe a Review Set of Doctors' Discharge Orders   Date: _____

★ HIGH PRIORITY

When you have completed Activity 20-2, take all the forms out of your chart. Your patient has been discharged! Your instructor will advise you of the proper procedure in preparing the patient's paper chart for transfer to the health information management department.

PHYSICIANS' ORDER SHEET 20-1

DATE	TIME	SYMBOL	ORDERS
			Case Manager to arrange for discharge planning
			Dr.

PHYSICIANS' ORDER SHEET 20-2

DATE	TIME	SYMBOL	ORDERS
			EKG today
			Repeat UA
			D/C Tobramycin
			PA & lat CXR DI: pre-DC
			D/C O$_2$, SVNs and IS-get ABGs in 2 hr
			D/C ES & US
			D/C ROM exercises
			Case Manager to arrange for DME——including
			walker & SVN machine
			Cardiac teaching prior to D/C
			Pt to be trans to Fajada Rehab Center in a.m.
			Please copy & send last 2 days of MAR, lab and x-ray
			results, & nursing & doctor's progress notes c̄ pt.
			Dr.
			D/C patient in a.m. after approved by Dr. Domonas
			Social service to arrange for transportation
			Dr.

Additional Transcription Practice (Samples of Pre-printed and Handwritten Doctors' Orders)

Included in Appendix A are sets of physicians' orders for medical and surgical patients. Many orders are of an advanced nature. They offer the student experience in transcribing handwritten and preprinted doctors' orders, and, perhaps most importantly, orders that have not been presented previously in this manual. The orders are rewritten from actual sets of doctors' orders obtained from hospitals and are representative of what the student will encounter on the job. If you use the Health Unit Coordinator Practice Activity Software for Transcription of Physicians' Orders, admit a new patient, create a new patient profile, or edit an existing patient's diagnosis in that patient's profile and transcribe the orders.

Sets of orders include:

A1-A8 provide practice transcribing doctors' orders covered in Chapters 10-18.

A9, A10 *A* and *B*, A11 *A* and *B*, and A12 *A-C* provide practice transcribing preprinted doctors' orders.

The orders A1-A8 are handwritten to provide students practice in interpreting doctors' handwriting and medical abbreviations. A typed interpretation of orders, including meaning of medical abbreviations, is included on the back of each set of orders. A typed version will not be available in the hospital, so try to interpret the orders from the handwritten orders prior to looking at the typewritten interpretation, provided on the following page of each set of orders.

PHYSICIANS' ORDER SHEET

DATE	TIME	SYMBOL	ORDERS
			Admit to Med Surg unit
			Dx: angina c dysrhythmia
			BRP only
			VS q4hr c orthostatics
			Soft diet
			Insert HL c rout. Na flushes
			EKG - LOC
			O₂ 2 L/min NP
			ASA 80 mg po now
			NTG 0.4 mg spray at BS
			Dr. Paul Rubenstein to
			consult and write addt'l
			orders ASAP
			Dr. Paul Miranda D.O.
			Start IVF of 5% D/H₂O 40 mEQ KCL @
			125 mL/hr
			Consent for heart cath c poss angioplasty
			+ Placement of stents
			Diazepam 15 mg IV on call to cath lab
			Dr. Paul Rubenstein MD
			T + X 2 units PC - hold
			Have consent signed for CABG
			Resp. to do preop teaching
			Valley anes to write pre op ord.
			Dr. Paul Rubenstein

A-1 Physicians' orders for a patient with a diagnosis of angina with dysrhythmia.

Admit to medical-surgical unit
Diagnosis: angina with dysrhythmia
Bathroom privileges only
Vital signs every 4 hours with orthostatics
Soft diet
Insert heplock with routine saline flushes
Electrocardiogram—leave on chart
Oxygen 2 liters per minute per nasal prongs
Aspirin 80 milligram per orally now
Nitroglycerin 0.4 milligram spray at bedside
Dr. Paul Rubenstein to consult and write additional orders as soon as possible
Dr. Frank Minard DO

Start intravenous fluids of 5 percent dextrose in water with 40 milliequivalent potassium chloride
    at 125 milliliter per hour
Consent for heart catheterization with possible angioplasty and placement of stents
Diazepam 15 milligram intravenous on call to catheterization laboratory
Dr. Paul Rubenstein MD

Type and crossmatch 2 units packed cells—hold
Have consent signed for coronary artery bypass graft
Respiratory (Cardiopulmonary) to do preoperative teaching
Valley anesthesia to write preoperative orders
Dr. Paul Rubenstein MD

			PHYSICIANS' ORDER SHEET

DATE	TIME	SYMBOL	ORDERS
			Admit to 4C — my service
			Dx: diabetes mellitus, gangrene lt foot
			Notify Valley anes of pt's adm
			Allergic to Tylenol & seafood
			ABR, ↑ lt foot on 2 pillows
			Foot cradle
			1500 cal ADA diet c̄ HS snack — FF
			Rout VS
			CMS lt foot q 2 hr
			Accu ✓ AC & HS
			Insert foley cath to st dr
			IVF of 0.45 NS 1000 mL c̄ 20 mEq KCl @ 125 mL/hr
			I & O
			Guaiac all stools, notify resident if +
			Levofloxacin 400 mg IVPB now, then 200 mg q day
			MS 10 or 12 mg q 3 — 4 hrs PRN
			Pepcid 40 mg PO BID
			Zolpidem 10 mg PO q HS
			Solu-Medrol 250 mg in 100 mL NS IV q 6 hrs,
			given over 1 hr, × 20 doses (total of 5 gms)
			Nurse practitioner to remain c̄ pt for first
			15 min of first infusion
			Eval time schedule for infusion to minimize
			sleep interruption
			Sliding scale with Humulin R: 250 - 299 - 5 units
			300 - 350 - 10 units, 351 - 399 - 15 units
			If > 399 call hospitalist
			Dr. Jason Federline MD

A-2 Physicians' orders for a patient with a diagnosis of diabetes mellitus, gangrene left foot.

Admit to 4C my service
Diagnosis: diabetes mellitus, gangrene left foot
Notify Valley anesthesia of patient's admission
Allergic to Tylenol and seafood
Absolute bed rest, elevate left foot on two pillows
Foot cradle
1500-calorie American Diabetic Association diet with bedtime snack—force fluids
Routine vital signs
Circulation, motion, and sensitivity left foot every 2 hours
Accu-check before meals and at bedtime
Insert Foley catheter to straight drainage
Intravenous fluids of 0.45 normal saline 1000 milliliter with 20 milliequivalent potassium chloride at
    125 milliliter per hour
Intake and output
Guaiac all stools, notify resident if positive
Levofloxacin 400 milligram intravenous piggyback now, then 200 milligram every day
Morphine sulfate 10 or 12 milligram every 3 to 4 hours as necessary
Pepcid 40 milligram per orally twice a day
Zolpidem 10 milligram per orally every bedtime
Solu Medrol 250 milligram in 100 milliliter normal saline intravenously every 6 hours, given over
    1 hour, times 20 doses (total of 5 grams)
Nurse practitioner to remain with patient for first 15 minutes of first infusion
Evaluate time schedule for infusion to minimize sleep interruption
Sliding scale with Humulin N; 250-299—5 units, 300-350—10 units, 351-399—15 units
If greater than 399, call hospitalist
Dr. Jason Federline MD

Consent for left foot amputation
Type and crossmatch two units packed cells—transfuse one—hold one
Valley anesthesia for preoperative orders
Dr. John Bamberl MD

PHYSICIANS' ORDER SHEET

DATE	TIME	SYMBOL	ORDERS
			Admit to ortho unit
			DX: MVA, contusions and abrasions fx rt Tibia
			@allergies: ASA, all dairy products
			BR c̄ rt leg immobilized c̄ sandbags
			VS q 4hrs until stable, then q shift
			mech soft diet
			Start IVF @ 1000 D₅/LR c̄ 20mg q MVI c̄ 100mL/h
			Ice bag to rt forearm
			ciprofloxacin 200 mg 1 IVPB q 12 hrs
			furosemide 40 mg IV push now then 20 mg q day
			chlorpromazine 25 mg now then 50mg IM q 4
			−6 hrs for N/V PRN
			Tylenol ī or ī̄ī PO q 4 hrs, for mild pain or discomfort
			oxycodone 30 mg PO q 6 hr for more sev. pain
			rabeprazole 20 mg PO q day after p̄ breakfast
			Temazepam 15 mg q HS PRN
			Dr. Melvin Cohen MD
			Consent for ORIF q Rt. Tibia
			Dr. Richard Davis for anesthesia
			Dr. Melvin Cohen MD
			MAY HAVE CL LIQ BREAK AT 0600, THEN NPO
			DEMEROL 120 MG @ 1000
			PHENERGAN 25 MG } IM
			Dr. Richard Davis MD

A-3 Physicians' orders for a patient with a diagnosis of motor vehicle accident, contusions and abrasions, fractured right tibia.

Admit to orthopedic unit
Diagnosis: motor vehicle accident, contusions and abrasions, fractured right tibia
Allergies: Aspirin, all dairy products
Complete bedrest with right leg immobilized with sandbags
Vital signs every 4 hours until stable, then every shift
Mechanical soft diet
Start intravenous fluids of 1000 milliliter 5% dextrose in lactated ringers with 20 milligrams of
    multivitamin at 100 milliliters per hour
Ice bag to right forearm
ciprofloxacin 200 milligram intravenous piggyback every 12 hours
furosemide 40 milligram intravenous push now, then 20 milligram every day
chlorpromazine 25 milligram now then 50 milligram intramuscular every 4 to 6 hours for nausea and
    vomiting as necessary
Tylenol 1 or 2 per orally every 4 hours for mild pain or discomfort
oxycodone 30 milligram per orally every 6 hours for more severe pain
rabeprazole 20 milligram per orally every day after breakfast
temazepam 15 milligram every bedtime as necessary
Dr. Melvin Cohen MD

Consent for open reduction, internal fixation of right tibia
Dr. Richard Davis for anesthesia
Dr. Melvin Cohen MD

May have clear liquid breakfast at 0600, then nothing by mouth
Demerol 120 milligram at 1000
Phenergan 25 milligram intramuscular

PHYSICIANS' ORDER SHEET

DATE	TIME	SYMBOL	ORDERS
			admit to IMC
			Dx: peritonitis
			NKA
			BRP c̄ help
			VS c̄ CVP q 2°
			Cardiac monitor
			NPO
			PICC with 1000 mg D₁₀/H₂O @ 120 ml/hr
			Foley to gravity with hourly output recorded
			Daily wt c̄ bed scale
			Measure abd girth q shift
			Replace tube as necessary
			NG tube to low cont suction
			cefaclor 250 mg IV q 8 hrs
			famotidine 40 mg q day
			zolpidem 30 mg q HS PRN
			MS 10 mg IM q 4-6 hrs for pain
			Tylenol #3 i-ii for H/A PRN
			Permit for laparotomy c̄ EUA
			Valley Anesthesia for pre-op orders
			Dr. H. Hogan DO
			Demerol (0.5mg) 0830AM
			Vistaril 25mg } IM
			Restoril 25 mg
			Clr liq breakfast at 0600, then NPO
			Dr. Peter Long MD

A-4 Physicians' orders for a patient with a diagnosis of peritonitis.

Admit to intermediate care
Diagnosis: peritonitis
No known allergies
Bathroom privileges with help
Vital signs with central venous pressure every 2 hours
Cardiac monitor
Nothing by mouth
Peripherally inserted central catheter with 1000 milliliter 10% dextrose in water at
    120 milliliter per hour
Foley to gravity with hourly output recorded
Daily weight with bed scale
Measure abdominal girth every shift
Rectal tube as necessary
Nasal gastric tube to low continuous suction
cefaclor 250 milligram intravenous every 8 hours
famotidine 40 milligram every day
zolpidem 30 milligram every bedtime as necessary
morphine sulfate 10 milligram intramuscularly every 4 to 6 hours for pain
Tylenol 2 per orally for headache as necessary
Permit for laparotomy with examination under anesthesia
Valley Anesthesia for preop order
Dr. Hy Hopes DO

Demerol 100 milligram at 0930
Vistaril 25 milligram intramuscularly
Restoril 15 milligram per orally bedtime
Clear liquid breakfast at 0600, then nothing per orally
Dr. Peter Fong MD

PHYSICIANS' ORDER SHEET

DATE	TIME	SYMBOL	ORDERS
			adm to med/surg
			Dx: gross hematuria — possible bladder CA
			Allergies: NKA
			Activity: as tol
			diet: reg
			VS: rout
			IVF ↓ 1000 mL LR @ 125 mL/hr
			strict I+O, urine output hourly
			Guaiac all stools
			labs: CBC, bmp, cea
			UA + culture
			Bld Cx x 2
			EKG — 20c
			Chest PA/Lat — eval for infiltrates
			Renal CT c̄ + s̄ contrast — poss malignancy
			total bone scan — mests
			Consent for: cystoscopy with bx
			per Dr. Peter Newma
			Oxycodone 5mg po every 4-6 hrs — severe
			pain
			acetaminophen ii PO hrs for H/A
			promethazine 25mg supp q 6 hr for N/V
			ciprofloxacin 250mg IVPB q 12 hrs
			Consult Dr. Robert Green — Oncology
			Dr. _____ MD
			Consent for Radical cystectomy
			Tx unit PC, Type 1 unit on hold for surg
			Dr Ross Kincaide for pre-op order — Dr. _____ MD
			NPO 2400 Demerol 100q ⟩ 0700
			Phenergan 25q ⟩ im
			Dr. _____ MD

A-5 Physicians' orders for a patient with a diagnosis of gross hematuria—possible bladder cancer.

Admit to medical surgical unit
Diagnosis: gross hematuria—possible bladder cancer
Allergies: no known allergies
Activity: as tolerated
Diet: regular
Vital signs: routine
Intravenous fluids: 1000 milliliter of lactated ringers at 125 milliliter per hour
Strict intake and output, urine output hourly
Guaiac all stools
Laboratory evaluations: complete blood cell count, basic metabolic panel, carcinoembryonic
   antigen
Urinalysis and culture
Blood culture times two
Electrocardiogram—leave on chart
Chest posteroanterior and lateral—evaluate for infiltrates
Renal computed tomography with and without contrast—possible malignancy
Total bone scan—metastasis
Consent for cystoscopy with biopsy
Dr. Peter Neuman

oxycodone 10 milligram per orally every 4 to 6 hours for severe pain
acetaminophen 2 per orally every 4 hours for headache
promethazine 25 milligram suppository every 6 hours for nausea and vomiting
ciprofloxacin 200 milligram intravenous piggyback every 12 hours
Consult Dr. Robert Goren - oncology
Dr. Philip Gormon MD

Consent for radical cystectomy
Type and crossmatch four units packed cells, transfuse one unit and hold three for surgery
Dr. Ross Kincade for preoperative orders
Dr. Robert Goren

Nothing by mouth 2400 hours
Demerol 120 milligram 0700 hours
Phenergan 25 milligram intramuscular
Dr. Ross Kincade MD

PHYSICIANS' ORDER SHEET

DATE	TIME	SYMBOL	ORDERS
			(handwritten orders)

A-6 Physicians' orders for a patient with a diagnosis of stage III breast cancer—asthma.

Admit to the service of Dr. Benjamin Robinowitz
Diagnosis: Stage III breast cancer—asthma
Activity: Up in chair as tolerated—bedside commode
Diet: regular as tolerated
Continuous intravenous fluids of 10% dextrose in water at 100 milliliter per hour
Intake and output
Daily weight at 0700 hours
Complete blood cell count, electrolytes stat
Complete metabolic panel in morning
Urinalysis
Chest x-ray anteroposterior and lateral—clinical indication: preoperative
Total bone scan—clinical indication: metastasis
Electrocardiogram
Pulmonary function tests
Arterial blood gases on room air and repeat in 1 hour after starting oxygen
Oxygen 2 liter per minute per nasal prongs
Thoracentesis with biopsy per Dr. Robinowitz
ampicillin 2 gram in 100 milliliter 5% dextrose in water intravenous piggyback every 6 hours
Advair inhaler 250/50—one puff two times a day
Singulair 10 milligram per orally every day
Tylenol number 1 (8 milligram of codeine) every 4 hours for pain
Valium 5 milligram for agitation every 6 hours as necessary
Bowel care of choice
Dr. Ryan Nash for oncology consult

Obtain computed tomography of chest done 1 week ago from Marycrest hospital
Dr. Paul Runion MD

Discontinue oxygen
Consent for total right mastectomy with implants
Dr. Benjamin Robinowitz MD

PHYSICIANS' ORDER SHEET

DATE	TIME	SYMBOL	ORDERS
			Post op ord Dr Sales post total
			mastectomy c̄ implant
			VS q 2° x 4, then q shift
			TCDB q 2° WA x 8°
			Keep hemovac comp Ice dry q shift
			Foley to st drainage
			Activity dangle feet out for 15', then
			up in chair for 20' then ↑ erc
			BR then bed rest hose
			Diet sips ↑ chips adv DAT
			Cont IVF @ 120 ml/HR (D5 ¼ R)
			IS q 2° x 8° then 6 x daily x 2 days
			IPPB c̄ 3 ml NS qID
			Daily H + H x 2 days
			DC bath in AM – st cath if
			unable to void in 6°
			Ampicillin 2 gm in 100 ml D5W
			IPPB q 6°
			Phenergan 25 mg q 6° prn N/V
			Demerol 50 mg IM q 4° pain
			Dr _____ MD
			BMP stat
			ABG stat
			O2 2 L/min per NP p̄ ABG
			Repeat ABG in 1 hr
			Dr Presta MD
			DC O2
			Convert IV to saline lock c̄ routine flushes
			Amb as tol
			Advair inhaler 250/50 1 puff BID
			Singulair 10 mg PO q PM
			Dr Benjamin _____ MD

A-7 Physicians' orders for a patient having had a total mastectomy with implants (postoperative orders)

Postoperative orders
Diagnosis: Status—post total right mastectomy with implants
Vital signs every 2 hours times 4, then every shift
Turn, cough, deep breath every 2 hours while awake times 8 hours
Keep Hemovac compressed and record drainage every shift
Foley to straight drainage
Activity: dangle this afternoon for 15 minutes, then up in chair for 20 minutes this evening
Bilateral thigh high Ted hose
Diet: sips and chips, advance diet as tolerated
Continue intravenous fluids at 120 milliliter per hour (5% dextrose in lactated ringers)
Incentive spirometry every 2 hours times 8 hours, then 6 times daily for 2 days
Intermittent positive pressure breathing with 3 milliliter normal saline four times a day
Daily hemoglobin and hematocrit for 2 days
Discontinue catheter in a.m. straight cath if unable to void in 6 hours
ampicillin 2 grams in 100 milliliter 5% dextrose in water intravenous piggyback every 6 hours
Phenergan 25 milligram every 6 hours for nausea and vomiting
Demerol 50 milligram intramuscular every 4 hours for pain
Dr. Benjamen Rabinowitz MD

Basic metabolic panel stat
Arterial blood gases stat
Oxygen 2 liters per minute per nasal prongs after arterial blood gases
Repeat arterial blood gases in 1 hour
Dr. Jason Resident MD

Discontinue oxygen
Convert intravenous to saline lock with routine saline flushes
Ambulate as tolerated
Advair inhaler 250/50—one puff two times a day
Singulair 10 milligram per orally every day
Dr. Benjamen Rabinowitz MD

PHYSICIANS' ORDER SHEET

DATE	TIME	SYMBOL	ORDERS
			Admit to medicine unit
			Dx: pneumonia c̄ hematemesis
			BR c̄ BSC
			Diet: mech soft as tol
			Insert HL with normal saline flushes
			I&O
			Chest PA/lat – CI: malignancy
			CT of chest c̄ and s̄ contrast
			Bronchoscopy c̄ Bx
			CBC, BMP, ESR stat PSA
			UA c̄ reflex
			Comp in am
			SVN c̄ Pulmicort 0.25 mg/2 ml of H_2O bid
			c̄ CPT
			Induced sputum spec to lab for gm stain and Cx
			ABG stat – call me with results of stat labs
			and bld abg
			Oxycodone 10 mg q 6 hr for pain
			Ambien 5 mg for sleep prn
			Dr Robert Sweet MD
			O2 @ 2 l/min and repeat abg in 2 hrs.
			Thoracentesis c̄ bx @ 0800
			Total bone scan - CI: metastasis
			Consultation c̄ Dr. John Pantwick
			Start PICC c̄ 0.45 NS @ 100 ml/hr.
			Ciprofloxacin 400 mg q 12 hrs.
			Dr. Robert Conner
			Consent for rt pneumonectomy
			Pt to return to surgical ICU postoperatively
			Pre op orders per Dr. Andrew Chung DO.
			Dr Robert Conner DO

A-8 Physicians' orders for a patient with a diagnosis of pneumonia with hematemesis.

Admit to medical surgical unit
Diagnosis: pneumonia with hematemesis
Bedrest with bedside commode
Diet: mechanical soft as tolerated
Insert heplock with routine saline flushes
Intake and output
Chest posteroanterior and lateral—clinical indication: malignancy
Computed tomography of chest with and without contrast
Bronchoscopy with biopsy
Complete blood cell count stat, basic metabolic panel, carcinoembryonic antigen stat
Prostate-specific antigen
Urine reflex
Comprehensive metabolic panel in a.m.
Small volume nebulizer with Pulmicort 0.25 milligram/2 milliliter of water two times a day with chest percussion therapy
Induced sputum specimen to laboratory for gram stain and culture
Arterial blood gases stat—call me with results of stat labs and blood gases
oxycodone 10 milligram every 6 hours for pain
Ambien 5 milligram for sleep as necessary
Dr. Robert Carver MD

Oxygen at 2 liter per minute and repeat arterial blood gases in 2 hours
Thoracentesis with biopsy at 0800
Total bone scan—clinical indication: metastasis
Oncology consult with Dr. John Pantavich
Start peripherally inserted central catheter with 0.45 normal saline at 100 milliliter per hour
ciprofloxacin 400 milligram every 12 hours
Dr. Robert Carver MD

Diagnosis: _FACIAL BURNS_____ Procedure _RHINOPLASTY FACIAL RECONS_

Comorbidities: ☐ Angina ☐ Atrial Fibrillation ☒ Cardiomyopathy ☐ COPD ☐ Congestive Heart Failure

☐ Diabetes with manifestations ☐ Diabetes, Insulin Dependent ☐ Diabetes, Uncontrolled ☐ Dehydration ☐ Malnutrition

Other ☐ _____

Consults:

☒ If any medical problems please call: Dr. _JEFF WEBER_____

☒ Additional Consults: _PAULA BROWNE_____

Activities:

☒ May be Out of Bed as desired when fully awake and reactive

☐ Additional Activities: _____

Treatments:

☒ Vital signs every 15 minutes until stable then every 4 hours   ☒ Encourage deep breathing and coughing

☒ Strict Intake and Output   ☒ If unable to void by __3 PM__ may use straight catheter

☒ Reinforce dressing as needed   ☐ If any surgical problems, please call me\

Diagnostics:

☒ _CONT. OXIMETRY_____ Reason _MONITOR O2 SATS_____

☐ _____ Reason _____

Medications:

☐ acetaminophen (325 mg) give 2 tablets (650 mg) orally every four hours as needed for mild pain (pain = 1-4)

☒ oxycodone/acetaminophen (Percocet) 5 mg/325 mg to be given orally every 4 hours as needed for pain:
　　　Moderate Pain (pain = 5 – 7) = 1 tablet
　　　Severe Pain (pain = 8 – 10) = 2 tablets

☒ ondansetron (Zofran) 4 mg slow IV push over 2 minutes **ONE TIME** for post op nausea. **Day of surgery only**

☐ prochlorperazine (Compazine): 5 mg slow IV every 6 hours as needed for nausea
　　　May give orally. **Total daily max dose: 40 mg**

1000 mL _RL_____ to infuse at __100__ mL/hr

Antibiotics Orders: _CEFADROXIL 250 mg I BID_____

Additional Orders: _DIGOXIN 0.125 mg/DAY_____

_JEFF WEBER_____

<u>Physician Name – Print and Sig – To Activate Only Orders Checked Above</u>　　Date　　　　　Time

_Jeff Weber MD_____

A-9 Preprinted physicians' orders for a patient with facial burns—scheduled for a rhinoplasty, facial reconstruction.

Diagnosis: Facial burns
Procedure: Rhinoplasty—Facial reconstruction
Dr. Jeff Weber
Additional consult: Paula Browne
Diagnostics: continuous oximetry—monitor oxygen saturation
1000 milliliter Ringers lactate to infuse at 100 milliliter per hour
Antibiotics Order: cefadroxil 250 milligram one twice a day
Additional Orders: digoxin 0.125 milligram per day
Dr. Jeff Weber MD

Diagnosis: _fx lt hip_

Comorbidities: ☐ Angina ☐ Atrial Fibrillation ☐ Cardiomyopathy ☐ COPD ☐ CHF ☐ Dehydration ☐ Malnutrition
☐ Diabetes with manifestations   ☐ Diabetes, Insulin Dependent   ☐ Diabetes, Uncontrolled
☐ Other: _____

Consults:
☒ Notify Primary Care Physician of admission

Treatments:
☒ Indwelling urinary catheter for hip fracture

Activity:
☐ Bedrest with 5# Bucks Traction for hip fracture.

Diet:
☐ Nothing by mouth
☒ Other: _cl liq – ADAT_

Diagnostics:
☒ Chest x-ray: Reason: _pre op_
☒ Arterial Blood Gases
☒ Electrocardiogram: Reason: _pre op_

Laboratory Requests:
☒ Complete Blood Count
☒ Partial Thromboplastin Time, Prothrombin Time
☒ Sodium, Potassium, Creatinine
☒ Urine reflex (reflex to culture if leukocyte or nitrite positive, also if moderate to many microorganisms found).
☒ Type & Screen.

Medications: Hold and Notify Physician of any Allergies to Ordered Medication.

☒ 1000 mL Dextrose 5% and 0.9% Sodium Chloride IV. Run at 75 mL/hour continuously.
☐ Add 20 mEq potassium chloride to each liter of IV fluids
☐ Other: _____
☒ Cefazolin Sodium (Ancef):1 gm IV piggyback: **Send with patient to Surgery**. Give every 8 hours for a total of 3 doses post op.
☐ Clindamycin 600 mg IV piggyback. Send with patient to Surgery. Give every 12 hours for 2 doses post op.
☒ **Notify physician if allergic to cephalosporins or penicillin**
☐ Other: _____
☒ Ondansetron (Zofran) 4 mg slow IV push over 2 minutes **one time dose** for post op nausea.**Day of surgery only**
☒ Prochlorperazine (Compazine) 5 mg slow IV push over 2 minutes every 6 hours as needed for nausea. May give orally
Total Maximum dose in 24 hours is 40 mg.

☐ Other: _____

Physician Name—Print and Sign—To Activate Only Orders Checked Above   Date   Time

M Peter... MD

Opportunity Medical Center

Orthopedic Hip Fracture
Order Set
Page 1 of 2   Rev 4/01/XX

[ORTHOHIP - 03282006]

A-10, A Page 1 of preprinted physicians' orders for a patient with a diagnosis of a fractured left hip (preoperative orders).

Medications Continued
Medications: **Hold and Notify Physician of any allergies to Ordered Medication.**

Pain Medications:

☒ Morphine Sulfate 2-10 mg to be given intravenously or intramuscular every 4 hours as needed for pain:
    Mild Pain (pain = 1-4) = 2 mg.
    Moderate Pain (pain = 5-7) = 4 mg.
    Severe Pain (pain = 8) = 8 mg.
    Severe Pain (pain = 9-10) = 10 mg.

☒ *If allergic to Morphine, give Meperidine and Hydroxyzine as indicated below, and discontinue Morphine.*
☒ Meperidine (Demerol) 25-100 mg given with Hydroxyzine (Vistaril) 25 mg **intramuscularly** every 4 hours as needed for pain:
    Mild Pain (pain = 1-4) = 25 mg Meperidine with 25 mg Hydroxyzine.
    Moderate Pain (pain = 5-7) = 50 mg Meperidine with 25 mg Hydroxyzine.
    Severe Pain (pain = 8) = 75 mg Meperidine with 25 mg Hydroxyzine.
    Severe Pain (pain = 9-10) = 100 mg Meperidine with 25 mg Hydroxyzine.

Choose ONLY ONE of the following narcotic and acetaminophen combination agents for moderate and severe pain management:

☐ Oxycodone/Acetaminophen (Percocet) 5 mg/325 mg 1-2 tablets to be given orally every 4 hours as needed for pain:
    Moderate Pain (pain = 5-7) = 1 tablet.
    Severe Pain (pain = 8-10) = 2 tablets.

☐ Propoxyphene/Acetaminophen (Darvocet-N 100) 100 mg/650 mg 1-2 tablets to be given orally every 4 hours as needed for pain
    Moderate Pain (pain = 5-7) = 1 tablet.
    Severe Pain (pain = 8-10) = 2 tablets.

☒ Acetaminophen (325 mg): Give two tablets orally every four hours as needed for mild pain (pain = 1-4) or fever > 101 degrees.
☐ Other: _____

Total Acetaminophen not to exceed 4 grams per day.

Additional Orders:

Hospitalist to √ Pt freq for pain ctrl.
VS q 4° hr til stable - call me if B/P > 190 or < 100
Pts husband may stay p̄ VS hours

Physician Name—Print and Sign—To Activate Only Orders Checked Above   Date   Time

Dr Pete Cng MD

Opportunity Medical Center

Orthopedic Hip Fracture
Order Set
Page 2 of 2   Rev 4/01/XX

[ORTHOHIP - 03282006]

A-10, B Page 2 of preprinted physicians' orders for a patient with a diagnosis of a fractured left hip.

on Page 1
Diagnosis: Fractured left hip
Diet: clear liquid—advance diet as tolerated
Diagnostics: Chest x-ray: Reason: preoperative
Electrocardiogram: Reason—preoperative

on Page 2
Hospitalist to check patient frequently for pain tolerance
Vital signs evey 4 hours until stable—call Doctor Ong if blood pressure greater than 190 or less
   than 100
Patient's husband may stay after visiting hours
Dr. Peter Ong MD

Diagnosis: _Ruptured disc—T3_   **Procedure:** ☐ Cervical ☐ Thoracic ☒ Lumbar ☐ Other_____

Admit Patient to : ☐ Critical Care ☒ Surgical Intermediate ☐ 5 C ☐ 2 B ☐ Other: _____

Comorbidities: ☐ Angina ☐ Atrial Fibrillation ☒ Cardiomyopathy ☐ COPD ☐ Congestive Heart Failure ☐ Dehydration ☐ Diabetes with manifestations ☐ Diabetes, Insulin Dependent ☐ Diabetes, Uncontrolled ☐ Malnutrition
☐ Other: _____

Consults:
☒ Fax Admission sheet to patients PCP: Dr _Linda Walker_
☒ Internal medicine doctor to see patient: Dr. _Harold Neuman to consult_
☒ Hospitalist to see and follow, please notify Dr. _pt. Hottelmeir_
☒ Physical Therapy consult
☐ Occupational Therapy Consult

Diet:
☐ NPO until fully awake
☐ Cold Liquids when alert
☒ Clear liquids: when alert. Then advance to patients normal diet as tolerated. _↓ Na_
☐ Ice chips and sips when fully awake

Activities:
☐ Bedrest   ☐ Head flat with one pillow   ☒ Elevate head of bed 15 degrees
☐ Elevate head of bed 30 degrees   ☐ Semi-sitting position
☐ Bathroom Privileges   ☐ Up as tolerated with LSO only
☐ Up to eat as tolerated   ☐ Up as tolerated

Treatments:
☒ Vital Signs and Neuro checks: ☐ Every 4 hours ☒ Every 1 hour X 2, every 2 hours X 4, then every 4 hours.
☒ Intake and Output
☒ If unable to void: may straight cath every 6-8 hours X 3. If still no void, anchor foley.
☐ Foley Cath to gravity.
☒ Incentive Spirometer every 2 hours while awake
☐ Oxygen 2 Liters per nasal cannula to maintain oxygen saturation greater than 93%
☒ Continuous pulse oximetry.
☐ Jackson Pratt drain to suction: Empty drain with sterile gloves. Compress bulb half-way. Record output every 4 hours.
☐ Sequential compression devices
☐ Cervical brace ☐ Soft cervical collar ☐ Miami J cervical collar ☐ Philadelphia Cervical Collar ☐ Other:_____
☒ Call _nurse_ _____ orthotics to fit for brace:
              Type: ☐ Hyperextension ☐ LSO ☒ TLSO ☐ Custom LSO ☐ Custom TLSO
☐ Abdominal Binder as needed

Laboratory: Do in AM:
☒ Complete Blood Count ☒ Basic Metabolic Profile ☒ Prothrombin time, APTT ☐ Urine Analysis

Medications: **Hold and Notify Physician of Allergies to Any Ordered Medication.**

☐ 1000 mL lactated ringers IV to run at _____ mL/hr

☒ 1000 mL dextrose 5% with 0.45% sodium chloride IV to run at 100 mL/hr

☒ Cefazolin (Ancef) 1 gm IV every 8 hours for a total of 3 doses.

☒ Ondansetron (Zofran) 4 mg IV slowly over 2 minutes for post op nausea **day of surgery only.**

☐ Prochlorperazine (Compazine) 5 mg IV over 2 minutes every 6 hours as needed for continued nausea.
     May give IM or orally. **Total maximum 24 hour dose = 40 mg**

☐ Trimethobenzamide (Tigan) 200 mg IM, orally, or rectally every 6 hours as needed for nausea

☐ Cyclobenzaprine(Flexeril) 10 mg: one tablet orally three times a day as needed for muscle spasms

☐ Diazepam (Valium) 5 mg orally every 6 hours as needed for muscle spasms

Physician Name— Print and Sign	Date	Time
Charles Wong MD		

Opportunity Medical Center

Spine Surgery- Johnson/Barrett
Post Operative Order Set
Page 1 of 2   Rev 4/01/XX

[SPINESURG - 08072006]

A-11, A Page 1 of preprinted physicians' orders for a patient having had surgery for a ruptured disc—third thoracic vertebra (postoperative orders).

Medications: **Hold and Notify Physician of Allergies to Any Ordered Medication.**

☐ Morphine sulfate 1-2 mg IV every 1 hour as needed for pain Notify Physician if pain not relieved after three doses of morphine or if Respirations are less than 15 / minute.
  Morphine 1 mg every 1 hours for moderate pain (pain= 5-7)
  Morphine 2 mg every 1 hour for Severe pain (pain = 8-10)

☒ Meperidine (Demerol) _75_ mg with hydroxyzine (Vistaril) _15_ mg Intramuscular every 3 hours as needed for pain.

☐ Codeine _____ mg with hydroxyzine (Vistaril) _____ mg intramuscularly every 3 hours for pain

☐ Acetaminophen 325 mg with oxycodone 5 mg (Percocet)1 -2 tablets orally every 4 hours as needed for pain.
  1 tablet for moderate pain (pain = 4-7)
  2 tablets for severe pain (pain = 8-10)

☐ Codeine 30 -60 mg orally every 2 hours as needed for pain
  Codeine 30 mg for moderate pain (pain = 4-7)
  Codeine 60 mg for severe pain (pain = 8-10)

☐ Acetaminophen 500 mg with Hydrocodone 5 mg (Vicodin) 1 to 2 tablets orally every 4 hours as needed for pain
  1 tablet for mild pain (pain = 1-4)
  2 tablets for moderate pain (pain 5-7)

☐ Acetaminophen 650mg with Propoxyphene (Darvocet N-100) 1 - 2 tablets orally every 4 hours as needed for pain.
  1 tablet for mild pain (pain = 1-4)
  2 tablets for moderate pain (pain 5-7)

☒ Acetaminophen 325 mg with Codeine 30 mg (Tylenol #3):Two tablets orally every 4 hours as needed for pain _mild_

☐ Acetaminophen 325 mg: 2 tablets (650 mg) orally as needed every 4 hours for mild pain or fever

Total Acetaminophen not to exceed 4 gms. per day.

Bowel Care of choice:
☒ Docusate sodium (Colace) 100 mg: one cap twice a day orally. Hold for loose stools.
☐ Milk of Magnesia (MOM) 30 mL orally daily as needed.
☐ Bisacodyl suppository (Dulcolax) 10 mg rectally as needed
☐ Fleets Enema (133 mL) rectally as needed
☐ Bisacodyl (Dulcolax) 5 mg orally as needed.

Additional Orders _Start Tomorrow —_
AVALIDE 300/12.5 mg ī q·DAY
PLAVIX 75mg ī q DAY
COREG 25 mg ī AM & HS
ZETIA 10mg ī HS
LIPITOR 40mg ī HS
Dr Harold Neuman for Cardio F/U

Physician Name—Print and Sign _Charles Wong MD_   Date   Time

Opportunity Medical Center

Spine Surgery- Johnson/Barrett
Post Operative Order Set
Page 2 of 2   Rev 4/01/XX

[SPINESURG - 08072006]

A-11, B Page 2 of preprinted physicians' orders for a patient having had surgery for a ruptured disc—third thoracic vertebra (postoperative orders).

on Page 1
Diagnosis: Ruptured disc—T3 (third thoracic vertebrae)
Primary care physician: Linda Valdez
Cardiologist: Gerald Neuman to consult
Notify Dr. Pat Stottolmeir
Advance to patient's normal diet as tolerated—low sodium
Call Sunrise orthotics to fit for brace

on Page 2
meperidine (Demerol) 75 milligram with hydroxyzine (Vistaril) 15 milligram
Start tomorrow:
Avalide 300/12.5 milligram 1 every day
Plavix 75 milligram 1 every day
Coreg 25 milligram 1 in the morning and 1 at bedtime
Zetia 10 milligram 1 at bedtime
Lipitor 40 milligram 1 at bedtime
Dr. Gerald Neuman for cardiovascular follow up
Dr. Charles Wong MD

Diagnosis: *Osteoarthritis torn meniscus*

Comorbidities: ☐ Angina ☐ Atrial Fibrillation ☐ Cardiomyopathy ☐ COPD ☐ CHF ☐ Dehydration ☐ Malnutrition
☐ Diabetes with manifestations • ☐ Diabetes, Insulin Dependent ☑ Diabetes, Uncontrolled
☑ Other *Chronic bronchitis - asthma*

Consults:
☑ Primary Care Physician: Dr. *Jared Jackson*
☐ Rehab Consult Dr. _____

Treatments:
☑ Incentive Spirometer every 1-2 hours while awake.
☑ Hemovac: record every shift. Remove Hemovac on Post op day _____.
☑ Change dressing on Post Operative day *2*.
☑ Indwelling urinary catheter. Remove catheter on Post Operative day _____
☑ If unable to void after Foley removed, scan bladder; May straight Cath for residual greater than 200 mL. May repeat if necessary one time. May re-insert Foley if continues. Notify physician in the morning of situation.
☑ Antiembolism hose:
Length: ☐ Knee ☑ Thigh
☑ Intake and output.
☐ Overhead frame, trapeze, bedboards
☐ Balanced Suspension.
☐ Routine Post Operative Vital Signs.
☐ Other: *SVN Q25 Ventolin 2M/NS q ll X 2days*

Activity:
Physical Therapy Consult.
Initiate Physician Protocol for:
☑ Total Knee Program: Occupational Therapy consult Post Operative Day 2.
☑ Continuous Passive Motion per protocol
☐ Special Weight Bearing Status. _____
Other: _____

Diet:
☑ Clear liquids to diet as tolerated when active bowel sounds present.
☐ Other: _____

Diagnostics:
Post Operative ☐ Right Knee ☑ Left Knee ☐ Do x-ray in PACU
Reason for x-ray: _____ ☐ Other diagnostics: _____

Laboratory Requests:
Hemoglobin and Hematocrit daily for two days
Sodium and Potassium daily for two days
☐ Daily Prothrombin Time
☐ Urine reflex when indwelling catheter removed. (Reflex to culture if nitrite or leukocyte positive or moderate to many microorganisms).
☐ Platelets every 3 days if on Enoxaparin *X 3*
☑ Other: *ABG on RA - call if results*

Physician Name—Print and Sign—To Activate Only Orders Checked Above   Date   Time

Jane Larasse NP

PATIENT IDENTIFICATION

Opportunity Medical Center

Ortho Post Operative Knee
Order Set
Page 1 of 3   Rev 4/01/XX

A-12, A Page 1 of physicians' preprinted orders for a patient having had a total left knee replacement (postoperative orders)

Medications:	Hold and Notify Physician of allergic medications ordered.

☒ 1000 mL dextrose 5 % with 0.45% sodium chloride IV at ☐ 20 _____ mL/hr continuous infusion.
☐ Add 20 mEq to each liter of IV fluids.
☐ 1000 mL dextrose 5% in Lactated Ringers IV at _____ mL/hr continuous infusion.
☐ 1000 mL dextrose 5% solution with 0.9% sodium chloride IV at _____ mL/hr continuous infusion.
☐ Convert IV to Saline Lock when tolerating fluids.
☒ Cefazolin Sodium (Ancef) 1 gram IV piggyback every 8 hours for a total of 3 doses
☐ Cefuroxime (Zinacef) 1.5 grams IV every 12 hours for 2 doses.
☐ Physician aware of penicillin allergy: OK to give cefazolin or cefuroxime
☐ Other: _____

☒ Morphine 2-10 mg Intravenous or intramuscular every 4 hours as needed for pain
    Mild Pain (pain = 1-4) = 2 mg
    Moderate Pain (pain = 5-7) = 4 mg
    Severe Pain (pain = 8) = 8 mg
    Severe Pain (pain = 9-10) = 10 mg

☒ **If allergic to Morphine give Meperidine and Hydroxyzine and discontinue Morphine**

☒ Meperidine (Demerol) and Hydroxyzine (Vistaril) **intramuscularly** every 4 hours as needed for pain
    Mild Pain (pain = 1-4) = Meperidine 25 mg and Hydroxyzine 25 mg
    Moderate Pain (pain = 5-7) = Meperidine 50 mg and Hydroxyzine 25 mg
    Severe Pain (pain = 8) = Meperidine 75 mg and Hydroxyzine 25 mg
    Severe Pain (pain = 9-10) = Meperidine 100 mg and Hydroxyzine 25 mg

Choose only one of the following oral agents for moderate and severe pain management

☐ Oxycodone 5 mg / Acetaminophen 325 mg (Percocet) 1-2 tablets, orally, every 4 hours as needed for pain
    Moderate Pain (pain = 5-7) = 1 tablet
    Severe Pain (pain = 8-10) = 2 tablets

☐ Hydrocodone 5 mg / Acetaminophen 500 mg (Lortab) 1-2 tablets, orally, every 4 hours as needed for pain
    Moderate Pain (pain = 5-7) = 1 tablet
    Severe Pain (pain = 8-10) = 2 tablets

☐ Propoxyphene 100 mg / Acetaminophen 650 mg, (Darvocet N-100), 1-2 tablets orally every 4 hours as needed for pain
    Moderate Pain (pain = 5-7) = 1 tablet
    Severe Pain (pain = 8-10) = 2 tablets

☒ Acetaminophen 325 mg : 2 tablets orally , every 4 hours, as needed for Mild Pain
          Total Acetaminophen not to exceed 4 grams per day.

☐ Warfarin (Coumadin) _____ mg orally today only.
☒ Warfarin (Coumadin): **Call for daily doses**
☐ Warfarin (Coumadin): Follow Scale for INR results:
    INR less than 0.9 : Give 5 mg
    INR 1.0 - 1.5 : Give 2.5 mg
    INR more than 1.6 : Give **NONE**
Other: _____

Physician Name- Print and Sign - To activate only orders checked above.	Date:	Time:
(signature)		

Opportunity Medical Center	Patient Identification
Ortho Post Operative Knee Order Set Page 2 of 3 Rev 4/01/XX	

A-12, B Page 2 of preprinted physicians' orders for a patient having had a total left knee replacement (postoperative orders).

Medications Continued

☐ Enoxaparin (Lovenox) 30 mg subcutaneous every 12 hours Start Date: ________ Time: ________
***If Creatinine Clearance is less than 30 mL/min **decrease dose to 30 mg DAILY**

☐ Enoxaparin (Lovenox) 40 mg subcutaneously **DAILY** Start Date: ________ Time: ________
*** If Creatinine Clearance is less than 30 mL/min **decrease dose to 30 mg DAILY**

☒ Ondansetron (Zofran) 4 mg slow IV push over 2 minutes **one time** for nausea **Day of Surgery only**

☒ Prochlorperazine (Compazine) 5 mg slow IV push over 2 minutes or intramuscularly every 6 hours as needed for nausea. May give Orally. **24 hour total maximum dose is 40 mg**

☒ Maalox ES 15 mL orally as needed for dyspepsia.

Choose one below for Bowel Care:

☐ Metamucil 1 packet mixed in fluid, orally, daily.
☒ Docusate 50 mg-Senna 8.6 mg: One tablet orally twice a day for bowel care
☐ Milk of Magnesia 30 mL orally as needed for bowel care
☐ Bisacodyl (Dulcolax) suppository 10 mg rectally as needed for bowel care
☐ Fleets enema: 130 mL as needed rectally for bowel care

Additional Orders:

May use rectal tube PRN - gas pains
On 3rd PO day start —
Advair 250/50 1 puff BID
Singulair 10 mg daily
Call if pt. shows any signs of SOB.

Physician Name — Print and Sign — To Activate Only Orders Checked Above	Date	Time
[illegible] MD		

PATIENT IDENTIFICATION

Opportunity Medical Center

Ortho Post Operative Knee
Order Set
Page 3 of 3 Rev 4/01/XX

A-12, C Page 3 of preprinted physicians' orders for a patient having had a total left knee replacement (postoperative orders).

on Page 1
Diagnosis: Severe arthritis—torn meniscus—left knee
Comorbidities: Chronic bronchitis—asthma
Primary care physician: Janet Jackson
Change dressing on postoperative day 2
Small volume nebulizer 0.25 (milliliter) Ventolin in 2 milliliter normal saline four times a day
    for 2 days
Hemoglobin and hematocrit very 4 hours three times
Arterial blood gases on room air—call with results

on Page 2
Intravenous at 120 milliliter per hour continuous infusion

on Page 3
May use rectal tube as necessary—gas pains
On third postoperative day start:
Advair 250/50 1 puff two times a day
Singulair 10 milligram every day
Call if patient shows any signs of shortness of breath
Dr. Paul Lacasse MD

APPENDIX B

Generic Hospital Forms and Examples of Downtime Requisitions That May be Used When Computers are not Available

PATIENT ACTIVITY SHEET

Room Number	Patient's Name	Activity

ADMISSION AGREEMENT (CONDITION OF ADMISSION)

Patient or someone acting for the patient agrees to the following terms of hospital admission.

1) **MEDICAL TREATMENT:** Patient will be treated by his/her attending doctor or specialists. Patient authorizes Hospital to perform services ordered by the doctors. Special consent forms may be needed. Many doctors and assistants (such as those providing x-rays, lab tests, and anesthesiology) may not be Hospital employees and are responsible for their own treatment activities.

2) **GENERAL DUTY NURSING:** Hospital provides only general nursing care. If the patient needs special or private nursing, it must be arranged by the patient or by the doctor treating the patient.

3) **MONEY AND VALUABLES:** The Hospital has a safe in which to keep money or valuables. It will not be responsible for any loss or damage to items not deposited in the safe. The Hospital will not be responsible for loss or damage to items such as glasses, dentures, hearing aids and contact lenses.

4) **TEACHING PROGRAMS:** The Hospital participates in programs for training of health care personnel. Some services may be provided to the patient by persons in training under the supervision and instruction of doctors or hospital employees. These persons may also observe care given to the patient by doctors and hospital employees. Photos or video tapes may be made of surgical procedures.

5) **RELEASE OF INFORMATION:** The Hospital may disclose all or any part of the patient's medical and/or financial records (INCLUDING INFORMATION REGARDING ALCOHOL OR DRUG ABUSE), to the following:

   a. **Third Party Payors:** Any person or corporation, or their designee, which is or may be liable under a contract to the hospital, the patient, a family member, or employer of the patient, for payment of all or part of the hospital's charges, including but not limited to, insurance companies, utilization review organizations, workman's compensation payors, hospital or medical service companies, welfare funds, governmental agencies or the patient's employer;

   b. **Medical Audit:** The Hospital conducts a program of medical audit and the patient's medical information may be reviewed and released by employees, members of the medical staff or other authorized persons to appropriate agencies as part of this program.

   c. **Medical Research:** Information may be released for use in medical studies and medical research.

   d. **Other Health Care Providers:** Information may be released to other health care providers in order to provide continued patient care.

   I understand that the authorization granted in items 5. a, b, c and d may be revoked by me at any time, except to the extent to which action has been taken in reliance upon it. The authorization will stay in effect as long as the need for information in items 5. a, b, c and d exist.

I have read and understand this Admissions Agreement, have received a copy and I am the patient, the parent of a minor child or the court appointed guardian for the patient and am authorized to act on the patient's behalf to sign this Agreement.

_____
WITNESS

_____
PATIENT   PARENT OF MINOR CHILD   COURT APPOINTED GUARDIAN
(PLEASE CIRCLE THE CORRECT TITLE)

_____
DATE   TIME

MEDICAL POWER OF ATTORNEY A.R.S. §14-5501: I appoint_____

_____
ADDRESS

_____
PHONE

as my agent to act in all matters relating to my health care, including full power to give or refuse consent to all medical, surgical and hospital care. This power of attorney shall be effective upon my disability or incapacity or when there is uncertainty whether I am dead or alive and shall have the same effect as if I were alive, competent, and able to act for myself.

_____
WITNESS

_____
PATIENT

FINANCIAL AGREEMENT

I agree that in return for the services provided to the patient, I will pay the account of the patient, and/or prior to discharge make financial arrangements satisfactory to the hospital for payment. If the account is sent to an attorney for collection, I agree to pay reasonable attorney's fees and collection expenses. The amount of the attorney's fee shall be established by the Court and not by a Jury in any court action. A delinquent account may be charged interest at the legal rate.

If any signer is entitled to hospital benefits of any type whatsoever under any policy of insurance insuring patient, or any other party liable to patient, the benefits are hereby assigned to hospital for application on patient's bill. However, IT IS UNDERSTOOD THAT THE UNDERSIGNED AND PATIENT ARE PRIMARILY RESPONSIBLE FOR PAYMENT OF PATIENT'S BILL.

IN GRANTING ADMISSION OR RENDERING TREATMENT, THE HOSPITAL IS RELYING ON MY AGREEMENT TO PAY THE ACCOUNT. EMERGENCY CARE WILL BE PROVIDED WITHOUT REGARD TO THE ABILITY TO PAY.

_____
PATIENT

_____
OTHER PARTY AGREEING TO PAY

_____
WITNESS

_____
RELATIONSHIP TO PATIENT

_____
DATE

PATIENT PROFILE (FACE SHEET)

1 PATIENT HOSP.NO.(M.R.#)	INFO STATUS		ACCOUNT NO. (BUS. OFF.)

2 PATIENT NAME LAST	FIRST	MIDDLE	ADM. DATE MO. / DAY / YR.	ADM. TIME	HOW BROUGHT TO HOSPITAL

3 PATIENT'S CURRENT ADDRESS STREET, P.O. BOX, APT. NO.	CITY	STATE	ZIP CODE	TELEPHONE NO.

4 PATIENT'S PERMANENT ADDRESS STREET, P.O. BOX, APT. NO.	CITY	STATE	ZIP CODE	TELEPHONE NO.

5 SEX 1. MALE 2. FEMALE	MARITAL STATUS 1. SINGLE 2. MARRIED 3. SEPARATED 4. DIVORCED 5. WIDOWED	RACE 1. WHITE 2. BLACK 3. INDIAN 4. ORIENTAL 5. OTHER	RELIGION 1. CATHOLIC 2. JEWISH 3. PROTESTANT 4. OTHER 5. LDS	AREA OF RESIDENCE

6 BIRTHDATE	AGE	PLACE OF BIRTH	MAIDEN NAME	SOC. SEC. NO./MEDICARE NO.

7 PATIENT'S OCCUPATION	UNION & LOCAL NO.	PATIENT'S EMPLOYER	ADDRESS	TELEPHONE NO.

8 PREVIOUSLY TREATED HERE? ☐ YES NAME ☐ NO USED	PREV. ADM. DATE MO. DA. YR.	PREV. ADMISSION 1. INPATIENT 2. OUTPATIENT	IF NEWBORN, MOTHER'S HOSP. NO.

9 UNIT	ROOM NO.	ACCOM. CODES 1. PRI 2. SEMI 3. NURSERY 4. PREMIE 5. ICU 6. RCU 7. CCU 8. VIP	ROOM RATE	PAY STATUS	CLASS OF ADMISSION 1. EMERGENCY 3. URGENT 2. ELECTIVE 4. OTHER

10 ADMITTING DIAGNOSIS

11 PHYSICIAN NAME	PHYSICIAN NO.	ADM. SERVICE	INFORMATION OBTAINED FROM:

12 SPOUSE OR NEAREST RELATIVE (NEXT OF KIN)	RELATIONSHIP	ADDRESS	TELEPHONE NO.

13 SECOND RELATIVE OR FRIEND	RELATIONSHIP	ADDRESS	TELEPHONE NO.

14 RESPONSIBLE PARTY NAME	RELATIONSHIP	SOC. SEC. NO.

15 RESP. PARTY ADDRESS STREET P.O. BOX APT. NO.	CITY	STATE	ZIP CODE	TELEPHONE NO.

16 RESP. PARTY OCCUPATION	NO. YRS. IN THIS EMPLOY	RESP. PARTY EMPLOYER	ADDRESS	TELEPHONE NO.

17 LENGTH OF TIME IN ARIZ.	1. OWN HOME 2. RENT HOME	TYPE OF HOME	BANK NAME & BRANCH	1. SAVINGS 2. CHECKING

18 CREDIT REFERENCES	1. NAME	ADDRESS	TELEPHONE NO.
19	2. NAME	ADDRESS	TELEPHONE NO.

20 INDUSTRIAL INJURY	DATE: MO. DA. YR.	CLAIM NO.	EMPLOYER'S NAME AND ADDRESS AT TIME OF INJURY

21 BLUE CROSS	NAME OF PLAN	GROUP NO.	IDENTIFICATION	EFFECTIVE DATE MO. DA. YR.	CITY	STATE

22 CHAMPUS DATA	PATIENT'S ID NO.	CARD EFFECTIVE MO. DA. YR.	CARD EXPIRES ON MO. DA. YR.	PATIENT OR SPONSORS BRANCH OF SERVICE	SERVICE CARD NO.
23	SPONSORS NAME	RANK-SERVICE NO.	DUTY STATION		

24 OTHER INSURANCE (INC. BLOOD BANK & BLUE SHIELD)	INS. CO. NO.	COMPANY NAME	POLICY HOLDER NAME	POLICY NO.	DATE ISSUED MO. DA. YR.	CITY	STATE
25	INS. CO. NO.	COMPANY NAME	POLICY HOLDER NAME	POLICY NO.	DATE ISSUED MO. DA. YR.	CITY	STATE

26 NAME OF HEALTH FACILITY DISCHARGED FROM WITHIN LAST 60 DAYS	ADDRESS

27 OTHER INFO.	V. A. ☐	COORDINATION OF BENEFITS ☐	INTERVIEWED BY	TYPED BY

28 REMARKS:

PHYSICIANS' ORDER SHEET

DATE	TIME	SYMBOL	ORDERS

GRAPHIC CHART

			A.M.			P.M.			A.M.			P.M.			A.M.			P.M.			A.M.			P.M.			A.M.			P.M.		
Date																																		
Hospital Days																																		
Day P.O. or P.P.																																		
HOUR			4	8	12 N	4	8	12 M	4	8	12 N	4	8	12 M	4	8	12 N	4	8	12 M	4	8	12 N	4	8	12 M	4	8	12 N	4	8	12 M		

Temperature/Pulse graph grid:

PULSE (Red)	TEMPERATURE (Black) F	C
	106°	41°
150	105°	
140	104°	40°
130	103°	
120	102°	39°
110	101°	
100	100°	38°
90	99°	
80	98.6°	37°
70	98°	
60	97°	36°
50	96°	35.5°

(• ORAL o RECTAL)

Respirations																																		
Blood Pressure																																		
Weight																																		

	7-3	3-11	11-7	Total	7-3	3-11	11-7	Total	7-3	3-11	11-7	Total	7-3	3-11	11-7	Total	7-3	3-11	11-7	Total
Intake Oral																				
Parenteral																				
Total																				
Output Urine																				
Drainage																				
Emesis																				
Total																				
Stools																				

GRAPHIC CHART

	PHYSICIANS' PROGRESS RECORD	
DATE	Note progress of case, complications, consultations, change in diagnosis, condition on discharge, instructions to patient.	

NURSES' NOTES AND ACTIVITY FLOW SHEET

DATE _____

INTAKE

IMED										
Solutions/ Amounts						BLOOD PRODUCTS	PO	TUBE FEEDING	FLUIDS PER TUBE	
Time	1/	2/	3/	4/	5/					
2400										
										2300-0700
8° Total	IV:									
Credit										
0800										
										0700-1500
8° Total	IV:									
Credit										
1600										
										1500-2300
8° Total	IV:									
Credit										24° TOTAL
24° Total	IV:									

OUTPUT

Time	Urine	Cath	N.G.	Emesis	C.T.		
2400							
8° Total							2300-0700
0800							
8° Total							0700-1500
1600							
8° Total							1500-2300
24° Total							24° TOTAL

BLOOD PRODUCTS

	UNIT #	TIME
1		
2		
3		
4		
5		
6		
7		
8		
9		
10		

SIGNATURES	
2300-0700	
0700-1500	
1500-2300	

CODES (EVALUATION/INTERVENTION)

1. NEW ORDER
2. DC'd, CATH INTACT
3. DRESSING CHANGED
4. TUBING CHANGED
5. ROUTINE SITE ROTATION
6. REDNESS AT SITE
7. SWELLING AT SITE
8. C/O PAIN
9. NO PROBLEM NOTED
10. OTHER (SEE NURSE'S NOTES)

IV MAINTENANCE RECORD

TIME	CODE	CATH SIZE	SITE	# STICKS	E/I	INITIALS

PATIENT RECORD-1

PATIENT NAME _____   DATE _____

	TIME									CODES
C A R D I O V A S C U L A R	HEART Intensity									
	RHYTHM									
	SKIN									
	COLOR									
	NAIL BEDS									
	CAPILLARY REFILL									
	EDEMA									
	RADIALS									
	PEDALS									
	TELEMETRY #									
	PACEMAKER Rate									
	Type/Mode									
G I	ABDOMEN									
	BOWEL SOUNDS									
	CIRCUMFERENCE									
N E U R O — COMA	EYES									
	VERBAL									
	MOTOR									
PUPILS RT	SIZE									
	REAC									
PUPILS LT	SIZE									
	REAC									
RT	ARMS									
	LEGS									
LT	ARMS									
	LEGS									
	FONTANEL									
R E S P I R A T O R Y	Respirations (Quality)									
	Breath RU									
	Sounds RL									
	LU									
	LL									
	O₂ MODE									
	Administration LF/FIO₂									
	SIGNATURES									

CODES

HEART INTENSITY
WNL- Within Normal
↓ - Muffled-Distant

RHYTHM
R - Regular
IR- Irregular

SKIN
W—Warm
C —Cold
H —Hot
DIA —Diaphoretic
MST—Moist
DR —Dry

COLOR and/or NAILBEDS
FL —Flushed
G —Good, Pink
P —Pale
DSK—Dusky
CY —Cyanotic
J —Jaundiced
ASH—Ashen
T —Tan

CAPILLARY REFILL
<3 seconds—Normal
>3 seconds—Sluggish
0—Absent

EDEMA
P —Pitting
NP—Non-pitting

PULSES
R/L
0 —Absent
1+ —Intermittent
2+ —Weak
3+ —Normal
4+ —Strong

TELEMETRY
NSR —Normal Sinus Rhythm
SB —Sinus Bradycardia
SVT —Supraventricular Tachycardia
PVC's —Premature Ventricular Contractions
AF —Atrial Fibrillation
VT —Ventricular Tachycardia
AIVR —Accelerated Idioventricular Rate
PAC's —Premature Atrial Contractions

PACEMAKER
Type:
PM—Permanent
TV —Transvenous
PW—Pacing Wires
Mode:
A—Asynchronous
D—Demand

ABDOMEN
FT —Flat
DIS —Distended
LG —Large
TEN—Tender
ST —Soft, Pliable
FM —Firm
RIG —Rigid

BOWEL SOUNDS
+ —Present
+o —Hypoactive
++ —Hyperactive
o —Absent

COMA SCALE
Eyes Open
4. Spontaneously
3. To speech
2. To pain
1. No response

Verbal Response
5. Oriented
4. Confused
3. Inappropriate
2. Incomprehensive
1. No response
C Crying

Motor Response
6. Obey commands
5. Localizes pain
4. Flexion-withdrawal
3. Flexion-abnormal (decorticate rigidity)
2. Extension to pain (decerebrate rigidity)
1. No response

PEDS COMA SCALE

Verbal Response		
>2 yrs	<2 yrs	
Oriented	Sociable	5
Confused	Consolable cry	4
Inappropriate	Persistent cry	3
Incomprehensible	Agitated	2
None	None	1

Best Motor Response		
Spontaneous	Appropriate for age	6
Localizes to pain		5
Withdraws to pain		4
Flexion to pain (decorticate)		3
Extension to pain (decerebrate)		2
No response		1

PUPIL REACTION
+ —Reacts
– —No reaction
c —Eye closed

PUPIL SCALE (mm)
1 2
3 4 5
6 7 8

ARMS & LEGS
6. Normal power
5. Mild weakness
4. Severe weakness
3. Spastic flexion
2. Extension
1. No response

RESPIRATIONS
R —Regular
I —Irregular
S —Shallow
L —Labored
RT —Retractions
STR—Stridor

FONTANEL
B - Bulging
F - Flat
SU—Sunken
P —Pulsing
T —Tense
SO—Soft

BREATH SOUNDS
CL—Clear
CR—Crackles
CS—Coarse
RA—Rales
RH—Rhonchi
W —Wheeze
I —Inspiratory
E —Expiratory
D —Decreased
0 —Absent

O₂ MODE
M —Mask
NP—Nasal Prongs
ET—Endotracheal
T —Trach
TN—Tent
H —Hood

PATIENT RECORD - 2

DATE _____

PATIENT CARE	2400						0800						1600						CODES
ISOLATION																			**ISOLATION** AFB—Respiratory BF —Blood & Body Fluids
TURN																			**TURN** R—Right L —Left B—Back
BATH																			**BATH** C —Complete P —Partial PA—Partial/Assist S —Shower SA—Shower/Assist SB—Self Bath T —Tub Bath TA—Tub Assist
ORAL/TRACH CARE																			
PERI/FOLEY CARE																			
ACTIVITY																			**ACTIVITY** BRPA— B —Bedrest A—AROM P—PROM H —Held PR —Playroom BRP —Bathroom Privileges BRPA—with assist BSC —Bedside Commode
BACK CARE																			
LINEN CHANGE																			
↑ SIDERAILS																			
																			BSCA—with assist C —Chair (Self) CA —with assist DA —Dangle/ Assist W —Walking WA —Walking/ assist S —Sleeping
DIET/APPETITE (% or cc's)																			
EQUIPMENT																			**RESTRAINTS** WRIST: left/right ANKLE: left/right BW —Both Wrists BA —Both Ankles P —Posey CC —Cadillac Chair CCA —with assist 2-3-4
GI TUBE — Placement Checked																			
GI TUBE — Tube type/ Suction																			
GI TUBE — Hematest, Color, Char.																			**DIET** FT—Fed Totally FP—Fed Partially TF—Tube Fed
STOOL — Method of Output																			**EQUIPMENT** IM —IMED OX—Oximeter KP—Kangaroo Pump AM—Apnea Monitor HO—Hypothermia Blanket
STOOL — Amt. Description																			HP—Hyperthermia Blanket A —Airshields Warmer
STOOL — Hematest																			IS —Isolette K —K-Pad
URINE — Catheter																			
URINE — Method of Output																			
URINE — Specific Gravity Color, Char.																			**STOOL/METHOD** T—Toilet D—Dilly I —Incontinent
RESP — Rx Chest Pt.																			
RESP — Suctioned																			**URINE/METHOD** Catheter Size/Date of Insertion D —Diaper BP—Bedpan I —Incontinent
RESP — Secretions (color, type, amt.) ET Oral																			
TESTS/PROC — Specimen Sent																			
TESTS/PROC — Procedures																			**PERI/FOLEY CARE** P—Peri F—Foley
TESTS/PROC — Tests/X-rays																			
DRAINS — Site Location																			**DRAINAGE** CL—Clear BL—Bloody S —Serous SS—Serosanguinous T —Tan
DRAINS — Dressing Change																			
WOUND — Site: location/ condition																			
WOUND — Dressing Change																			
FLAPS/GRAFTS																			
SIGNATURES																			

PATIENT RECORD - 3

PATIENT NAME _____   DATE _____

NOTIFICATION	TIME	NURSING CONCERNS	RESPONSE TIME/ACTION TAKEN	INIT.

DISCHARGE/TEACHING INSTRUCTIONS

PATIENT BEHAVIORS/OBSERVATIONS/EVALUATION/INTERVENTIONS (NURSES' NOTES)

PATIENT RECORD - 4

HISTORY AND PHYSICAL EXAMINATION

Final Diagnosis: To be recorded when determined_____

_____

Age____Sex_____Race____S.M.W. yrs. ____ Adm. ____ Dis. ____

_____

Family History	Age	Health, if living, or cause of death Note especially Hereditary or Infectious diseases
Father		
Mother		
Brothers		
Sisters		

Chief Complaint: Date and mode of onset, probable cause, course

Past History: Diseases from childhood to date, habits, menstrual history, social data_____

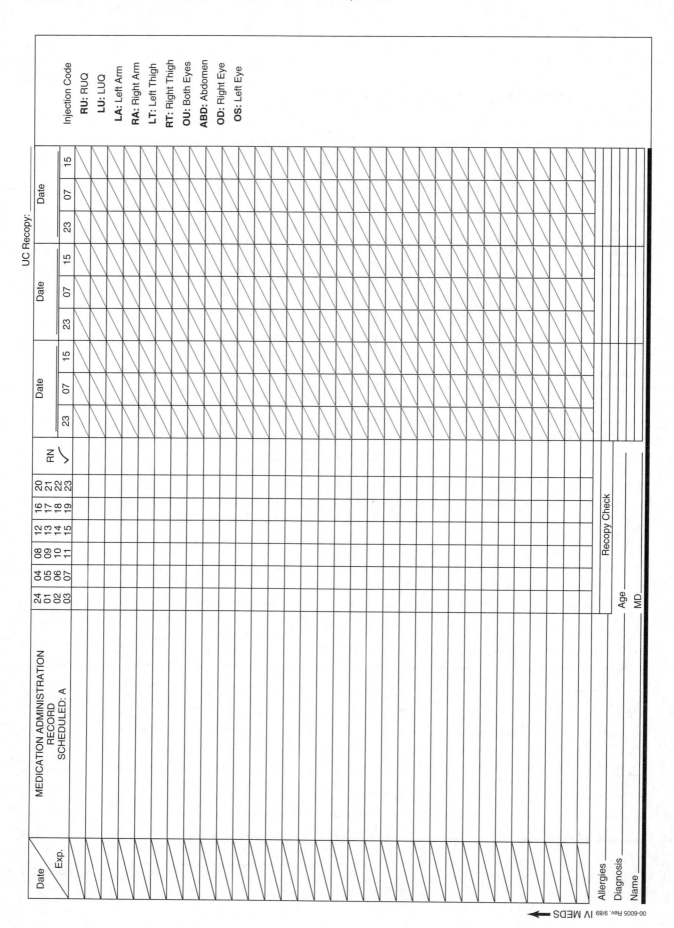

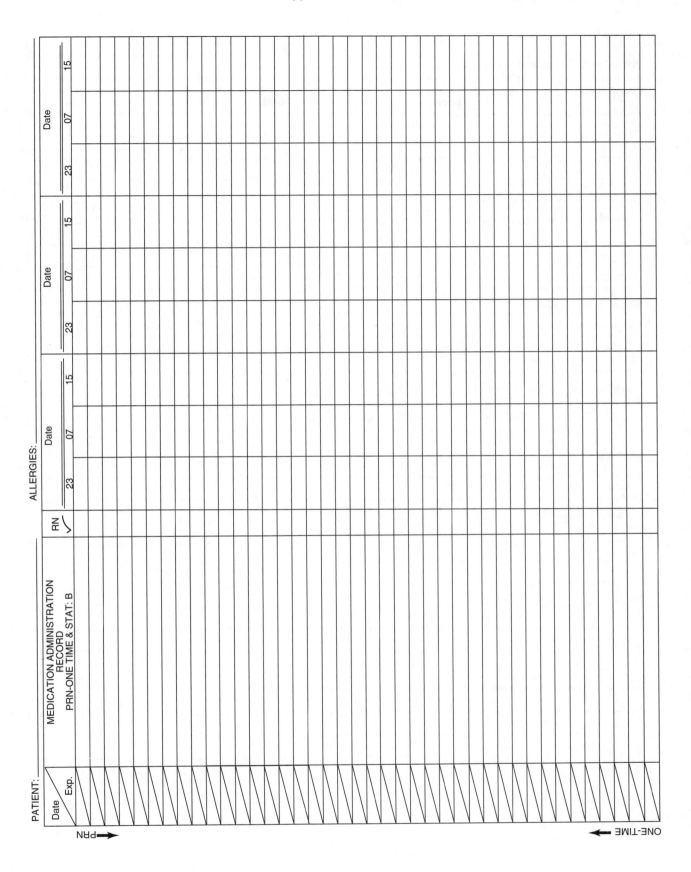

PHYSICIANS' DISCHARGE SUMMARY

Patient Name: _____

MR#: _____

Date of Admission: _____

Date of Discharge: _____

Principle Diagnosis: _____

_____

_____

_____

Secondary Diagnosis: _____

_____

_____

_____

Operations or Procedures:

_____

_____

_____

Brief History and Essential Physical Findings:

_____

_____

_____

_____

_____

Significant Laboratory, X-ray and Consultation Findings:

_____

_____

_____

Course in Hospital with Complications, if any:

_____

_____

Disposition including follow-up treatment, medication by name and dosage, discharge instructions:

_____

_____

_____

_____

_____

_____

Physician's Signature: _____

NURSES' DISCHARGE PLANNING INSTRUCTIONS

DATES OF HOSPITALIZATION   FROM_____TO_____ DISCHARGE DATE_____ TIME _____

HOSPITAL DIAGNOSIS: **1.**_____   **2.**_____

3._____   **4.**_____

DIET INSTRUCTIONS:_____

TREATMENTS:_____

ACTIVITIES:_____

SUPPLIES:_____

MEDICATIONS	STRENGTH	INSTRUCTIONS	PRESCRIPTION GIVEN	
			YES	NO
1.				
2.				
3.				
4.				
5.				
6.				
7.				
8.				

CALL DR._____ OFFICE FOR APPOINTMENT IN/ON_____ _____M.D.

I UNDERSTAND THE ABOVE INSTRUCTIONS   YES ☐   NO ☐   ALL PERSONAL BELONGINGS TAKEN HOME   YES ☐   NO ☐

IF NO EXPLAIN_____

DATE_____ TIME_____ PATIENT/RESPONSIBLE PARTY SIGNATURE _____

INDEPENDENT IN ADL   YES ☐   NO ☐   ALERT ☐   ORIENTED TO TIME AND PLACE ☐   DISORIENTED ☐

CONFUSED: AT INTERVALS ☐   AT NIGHT ONLY ☐   SEMI-COMATOSE ☐   COMATOSE ☐

DESCRIPTION OF SKIN _____

DESCRIPTION OF INCISION _____

BRIEFLY DESCRIBE ANY PROBLEM IN THE FOLLOWING AREAS:

VISION_____ HEARING _____ SPEECH_____

AMBULATION_____ DEFORMITY_____ PROSTHESIS/ EQUIPMENT_____

OTHER _____

MODE OF DISCHARGE _____ ACCOMPANIED BY_____ DISCHARGE DESTINATION_____

HOME CARE REFERRAL: NO_____YES_____AGENCY_____

DATE _____ RN _____

MR 685-755 (T) REV. 5-80

DISCHARGE INSTRUCTIONS   CHART COPY

HEALTH UNIT COORDINATOR / HEALTH UNIT COORDINATOR PROCEDURES

ROUTINES AND TESTS / KARDEX

GateWay Community College

		PAST MEDICAL HISTORY	X-RAY OTHER PROCEDURES	DATE ORD.	DATE TO BE DONE	DAILY LAB	DATE ORD		ALLERGIES

ACTIVITY — AD LIB-WALK-CHAIR-BRP-BR

TREATMENTS

CONSULTANTS

VITALS — TIME

WEIGHT

DIET — LAB — DATE ORD. — DATE TO BE DONE — DATE ORD — SOCIAL SERV/CASE MGR

Tube Feedings — PHYSICAL MEDICINE

SPECIMENS

P.I.V. — URINE

FLUID BALANCE — SPUTUM — RESP. THER (CARIO PULM)

Central Line — STOOL — O₂

Invasive lines (eg. Arterial, CVP) — OTHER — TREATMENTS

BLOOD GLUC MONIT

NG — SURGERIES — TRACTION/ORTHO — OTHER

I & O

FOLEY

DIAGNOSIS _____   ADMITTING PHYSICIAN _____   CODE STATUS _____

PATENT NAME _____   ADMISSION DATE _____   ROOM # _____

JMP Medical Center

HEALTH UNIT COORDINATOR
HEALTH UNIT COORDINATOR PROCEDURES

Patient Label

Doctor ordering _____

Today's date _____

Requested by _____

NUTRITIONAL CARE DEPARTMENT REQUISITION

- ☐ Bland
- ☑ Soft 1500 Calorie ADA
- ☐ Clear liquid
- ☐ Dysphagia _____
- ☐ Finger food
- ☐ Force fluids
- ☐ Full liquid
- ☐ Gluten free
- ☐ Kosher
- ☐ Low cholesterol
- ☐ Low sodium

- ☐ Mechanical soft
- ☐ Modified fat
- ☐ Pediatric
- ☐ Protein modified _____ g
- ☐ Prudent cardiac
- ☐ Pureed
- ☐ Regular
- ☐ Renal
- ☐ Restrict Fluids to _____
- ☐ Snacks / supplements
- ☐ _____ Sodium

- ☐ Soft
- ☐ Tube Feeding _____

- ☐ Vegetarian
- ☐ Calorie count
- ☐ Dietitian consult
- ☐ Early tray
- ☐ Guest tray
- ☐ Hold tray
- ☐ NPO
- ☐ Release from hold

- ☐ Other _____

Food Allergies _____

Preferences _____

Comments _____

JMP Medical Center

HEALTH UNIT COORDINATOR
HEALTH UNIT COORDINATOR PROCEDURES

Doctor ordering _____   ☐ Stat
Today's date _____   ☐ Timed
Draw @ date _____ Time _____   ☐ Routine
Collection date _____ Time _____
Collected by _____
Requested by _____

☐ Patient Label

Hematology, Serology, & Urinalysis / Urine Chemistry Requisition

Hematology	**Serology**	**Urinalysis / Urine Chemistry**
☐ Bleeding time, Ivy	☐ ANA	☐ Routine UA
☐ CBC c̄ diff	☐ ASO titer	☐ Reflex UA
☐ CBC c̄ manual diff	☐ CEA	☐ Amylase (2hr)
☐ Factor VIII	☐ CMV	☐ Bilirubin
☐ Fibrinogen	☐ IgG	☐ Calcium
☐ HCT	☐ IgM	☐ Chloride
☐ HGB	☐ Cocci screen	☐ Creatinine clearance 24 hour
☐ H & H	☐ EBV panel	☐ Glucose tolerance
☐ Eosinophil Ct absolute	☐ Enterovirus Ab panel 1	☐ Nitrogen
☐ Eosinophil smear	☐ Enterovirus Ab panel 2	☐ Occult blood
☐ ESR	☐ FTA	☐ Osmolality
☐ LE cell prep	☐ Hepatitis screen	☐ Phosphorus
☐ Platelet Ct	☐ HbsAb	☐ Potassium
☐ PT/INR	☐ HbsAg	☐ Pregnancy
☐ PTT (APTT)	☐ HIV	☐ Protein
☐ RBC	☐ Monospot	☐ Sodium
☐ RBC Indices	☐ Methodology _____	☐ Sp gravity
☐ Reticulocyte Ct	☐ PSA screen	☐ Uric Acid
☐ Sickle cell prep	☐ RA factor	☐ Other
☐ WBC	☐ RPR	
☐ WBC c̄ diff	☐ RSV	
☐ WBC c̄ manual diff	☐ Rubella screen	
☐ Other	☐ Streptozyme	

☐ Write in item _____

_____

JMP Medical Center

HEALTH UNIT COORDINATOR
HEALTH UNIT COORDINATOR PROCEDURES

Doctor ordering _____ ☐ Stat

Today's date _____ ☐ Timed

Draw @ date _____ Time _____ ☐ Routine

Requested by _____

| Patient Label |

CHEMISTRY & TOXICOLOGY REQUISITION

CHEMISTRY	CHEMISTRY CONT'D	TOXICOLOGY
Panels	*Tests cont'd*	
☐ Electrolytes	☐ Cortisol	☐ Acetaminophen
☐ BMP	☐ Ferretin	☐ Peak
☐ CMP	☐ Folic Acid	☐ Trough
☐ Renal	☐ Folate	☐ Aminophylline
☐ Hepatic	☐ FSH	☐ Peak
☐ Lipid	☐ Glucose	☐ Trough
Tests	☐ Glucose _____ Hr PP	☐ Digitoxin
☐ Acetone	☐ Glucose Tolerance	☐ Peak
☐ Ace Level	☐ Iron	☐ Trough
☐ ACTH	☐ Lactic Acid	☐ Dilantin
☐ A/G Ratio	☐ LDH	☐ Peak
☐ Albumin	☐ LH	☐ Trough
☐ Aldolase	☐ Lipase	☐ Drug Screen
☐ Alk Phos	☐ Magnesium	☐ ETOH/alcohol
☐ Amylase	☐ Osmolality	☐ Gentamycin
☐ ALT (SGPT)	☐ Osmolarity	☐ Peak
☐ AST (SGOT)	☐ Phosphorous	☐ Trough
☐ Bilirubin, total	☐ Potassium	☐ Kanamycin
☐ Direct	☐ Protein	☐ Peak
☐ Indirect	☐ Protein Electrophoresis	☐ Trough
☐ BNP	☐ Sodium	☐ Lidocaine
☐ BUN	☐ TBG	☐ Peak
☐ Calcium	☐ TIBC	☐ Trough
☐ Carbon Dioxide	☐ Triglycerides	☐ Phenobarbital
☐ Chloride	☐ Troponin	☐ Peak
☐ Cholesterol	☐ TSH	☐ Trough
☐ Citrate	☐ T_3	☐ Tobramycin
☐ CK (CPK)	☐ T_4	☐ Peak
☐ CKMB	☐ Uric Acid	☐ Trough
☐ C-reactive protein	☐ VMA	☐ Vancomycin
☐ Creatinine		☐ Peak
		☐ Trough

☐ Write in item _____

JMP Medical Center

HEALTH UNIT COORDINATOR
HEALTH UNIT COORDINATOR PROCEDURES

Doctor ordering _____ ☐ Stat

Today's date _____ ☐ Timed

Collection date _____ Time _____ ☐ Routine

Collected by _____

Requested by _____

Patient Label

Antibiotics: _____

MICROBIOLOGY, FLUIDS, & CYTOLOGY REQUISITION

Microbiology

Specimen Source
- ☐ Abscess
  _____
- ☐ Blood
- ☐ Body Cavity
  _____
- ☐ CSF
- ☐ Ear Drainage
  - ☐ Right
  - ☐ Left
- ☐ Eye Drainage
  - ☐ Right
  - ☐ Left
- ☐ Nasal Smear
- ☐ Sputum
- ☐ Stool
- ☐ Throat
- ☐ Tissue
  _____
- ☐ Urine
  - ☐ Voided
  - ☐ Clean Catch
  - ☐ St Cath
  - ☐ Foley Cath
- ☐ Wound Drainage _____
- ☐ Other _____

Test Requested
- ☐ AFB Culture
- ☐ AFB Stain
- ☐ C & S
- ☐ C & S Anaerobic
- ☐ C. Diff
- ☐ Fungal Culture
- ☐ GC Screen
- ☐ G-Stain
- ☐ Strep Screen
- ☐ Viral Culture
- ☐ Other
  _____
- ☐ Stool
  - ☐ Fat
  - ☐ Fiber
  - ☐ Occult Blood
  - ☐ Ova & Parasites
    - ☐ #1 of 3
    - ☐ #2 of 3
    - ☐ #3 of 3

Fluids

Specimen Source
- ☐ Abdominal
- ☐ Amniotic
- ☐ CSF
- ☐ Pericardial
- ☐ Peritoneal
- ☐ Pleural
- ☐ Synovial
- ☐ Other
- # of Tubes _____

Test Requested
- ☐ Cell Count c̄ diff
- ☐ Glucose
- ☐ LDH
- ☐ Occult Blood
- ☐ Protein
- ☐ Sp Gravity
- ☐ RPR (CSF)
- ☐ Micro
  _____
- ☐ Other
  _____

Cytology

Specimen Source
- ☐ Amniotic
- ☐ Breast Bx
- ☐ Bronchial Asp
- ☐ Buccal
- ☐ Cervical Smear
- ☐ Cervical Bx
- ☐ Colon Bx
- ☐ CSF
- ☐ Gastric Fluid
- ☐ Lung Asp
- ☐ Pleural
- ☐ Pericardial
- ☐ Peritoneal
- ☐ Sputum
- ☐ Vaginal
- ☐ Other

Test Requested
- ☐ Pap
- ☐ Fungal
- ☐ Maturation Index
- ☐ Other
  _____

JMP Medical Center

HEALTH UNIT COORDINATOR
HEALTH UNIT COORDINATOR PROCEDURES

Patient Label

Doctor ordering _____ ☐ Stat
Today's date _____ ☐ Routine
Collection date _____ Time _____
Collected by _____
Requested by _____

BLOOD BANK REQUISITION

☐ Routine   ☐ ASAP   ☐ Stat   ☐ For Hold

Date of Surgery _____   Date of Transfusion _____

Autologous Blood? ☐ Yes ☐ No   ☐ Whole Blood _____ # of Units
Donor Specific? ☐ Yes ☐ No   ☐ Packed Cells _____ # of Units
☐ Type and X-match   ☐ Washed Cells _____ # of Units
☐ Type and Screen   ☐ Granulocytes _____ # of Units
                                       ☐ Fresh Frozen Plasma _____ # of Units
☐ Coombs' Test   ☐ Platelet Concentrate _____ # of Units
☐ Other _____   ☐ Cryoprecipitate _____ # of Units
                                       ☐ Other _____

Comments _____
_____
_____

CONSENT FOR TRANSFUSION(S)

1. I authorize the administration of such transfusions of whole blood or blood products to the above patients as may be deemed advisable in the judgment of the patient's attending physician, his associates or assistants.

2. It has been fully explained to me and I understand that blood transfusions are not always successful in producing a desirable result. It has also been explained to me and I understand that despite the exercise of due care, the transfusion of blood or blood products is always attended with a possibility of some ill effects, such as: the transmission of hepatitis; accidental immunization; allergic reactions; or in rare instances Acquired Immune Deficiency Syndrome (AIDS).

3. It has also been explained to me and I understand that emergencies do, on occasion, arise when it may be necessary for the patient's well being to use existing stocks of blood which may not include the most compatible blood types.

4. **I UNDERSTAND AND AGREE THAT NO GUARANTEE OR WARRANTY (INCLUDING THE IMPLIED WARRANTIES OF MERCHANTABILITY AND FITNESS) APPLIES TO THE BLOOD OR BLOOD PRODUCTS WHICH MAY BE SUPPLIED TO THIS PATIENT.**

5. I accept on behalf of this patient all of the risks referred to above.

_____   _____
       Patient   **Witness**

_____   _____
  Person Authorized to Sign for Patient   **Date**

_____
      Relationship

_____

Reason for signature by person authorized to sign for patient in lieu of, or in addition to, signature by patient.

Consent For Transfusion Of Blood Or Blood Products

1. I HAVE BEEN INFORMED that I need or may need during treatment, a transfusion of blood and/or one of its products in the interest of my health and proper medical care.

2. I HAVE BEEN INFORMED of the risks and benefits of receiving transfusion(s). These risks exist despite the fact that the blood has been carefully tested.

3. The alternatives to transfusion, including the risks and consequences of not receiving this therapy, have been explained to me.

4. I have read, or had read to me, the Blood Transfusion Information regarding blood transfusions and have had the opportunity to ask questions.

5. I hereby consent to the transfusion(s).

Patient's Signature	Date	Time

Signature of parent, legally appointed guardian or responsible person
(for patients who cannot sign)

Witness	Date	Time

Refusal To Permit Blood Transfusion

1. I request that no blood derivatives be administered to _____
   during this hospitalization.   (patient name)

2. I hereby release the hospital, its personnel and the attending physician from any responsibility whatever for unfavorable reactions or any untoward results due to my refusal to permit the use of blood or its derivatives.

3. I fully understand the possible consequences of such refusal on my part.

_____   _____   _____
Patient's Signature   Date   Time

Signature of parent, legally appointed guardian or responsible person
(for patients who cannot sign)

_____   _____   _____
Witness   Date   Time

_____   _____   _____
Witness   Date   Time

HEALTH UNIT COORDINATOR
HEALTH UNIT COORDINATOR PROCEDURES

JMP Medical Center

Patient Label

Doctor ordering ✓ for infiltrates, acute abd., tumor

Today's date March 30/19

Date to be done March 31/19

☐ Stat   ☑ Routine   ☐ ASAP

Requested by _____

RADIOGRAPHIC (X-RAY) PROCEDURES REQUISITION

Clinical indication

Transportation   ☐ Portable   ☐ Stretcher   ☑ Wheelchair   ☐ Ambulatory

O₂   ☐ Yes / ☑ No   Diabetic ☐ Yes / ☑ No
IV   ☐ Yes / ☑ No   Seizure disorder ☐ Yes / ☑ No
Isolation ☐ Yes / ☑ No   Non-English speaking ☐ Yes / ☑ No

Write out the entire doctor's order

Comments _____

Hearing deficit ☐ Yes / ☑ No
Sight deficit ☐ Yes / ☑ No

☐ Abdomen
☐ Bone age study
☐ Bone x-ray order
☑ Chest order
☐ IVP/IVU
☑ KUB / flat plate of abdomen
☑ Mammogram
☐ Sinus series order
☐ SNAT series
☐ Spine order
☐ BE
☐ SBFT
☐ UGI
☐ Write in order

HEALTH UNIT COORDINATOR
HEALTH UNIT COORDINATOR PROCEDURES

JMP Medical Center

Patient Label

Doctor ordering _____

Today's date _____ ☐ Stat ☐ Routine ☐ ASAP

Date to be done _____ Requested by _____

SPECIAL INVASIVE X-RAY PROCEDURES REQUISITION

Clinical indication _____

Transportation ☐ Portable ☐ Stretcher ☐ Wheelchair ☐ Ambulatory

O₂ ☐ Yes / ☐ No Diabetic ☐ Yes / ☐ No Hearing deficit ☐ Yes / ☐ No

IV ☐ Yes / ☐ No Seizure disorder ☐ Yes / ☐ No Sight deficit ☐ Yes / ☐ No

Isolation ☐ Yes / ☐ No Non-English speaking ☐ Yes / ☐ No

Write out the entire doctor's order _____

Comments _____

☐ Angiogram _____

☐ Arteriogram _____

☐ Arthrogram _____

☐ Cervical myelogram _____

☐ Cholangiogram _____

☐ Hysterosalpingogram _____

☐ Lymphangiogram _____

☐ PTHC _____

☐ Spinal myelogram _____

☐ Venogram _____

☐ Voiding cystourethrogram _____

☐ Write in order _____

JMP Medical Center

HEALTH UNIT COORDINATOR
HEALTH UNIT COORDINATOR PROCEDURES

Patient Label

Doctor ordering _____

Date to be done _____   ☐ Stat   ☐ Routine   ☐ ASAP

Today's date _____   Requested by _____

COMPUTED TOMOGRAPHY REQUISITION

Clinical indication
☐ With contrast   ☐ Without contrast

Transportation   ☐ Portable   ☐ Stretcher   ☐ Wheelchair   ☐ Ambulatory

O₂   ☐ Yes / ☐ No
IV   ☐ Yes / ☐ No
Isolation   ☐ Yes / ☐ No

Diabetic   ☐ Yes / ☐ No
Seizure disorder   ☐ Yes / ☐ No
Non-English speaking ☐ Yes / ☐ No

Hearing deficit   ☐ Yes / ☐ No
Sight deficit   ☐ Yes / ☐ No

Write out the entire doctor's order

Comments _____

☐ CT scan of head _____
☐ CT scan of brain _____
☐ CT scan of abdomen _____
☐ CT scan of pelvis _____
☐ CT scan of spine _____
☐ CT of neck _____
☐ CT-guided liver biopsy _____
☐ DSA (digital subtraction angiogram) _____
☐ 64 Slice cardiac CT _____
☐ Write in order _____

JMP Medical Center

HEALTH UNIT COORDINATOR
HEALTH UNIT COORDINATOR PROCEDURES

Patient Label

Doctor ordering _____

Today's date _____   ☐ Stat   ☐ Routine   ☐ ASAP

Date to be done _____   Requested by _____

ULTRASONOGRAPHY REQUISITION

Clinical indication

Transportation   ☐ Portable   ☐ Stretcher   ☐ Wheelchair   ☐ Ambulatory

O₂   ☐ Yes / ☐ No
IV   ☐ Yes / ☐ No
Isolation   ☐ Yes / ☐ No

Diabetic   ☐ Yes / ☐ No
Seizure disorder   ☐ Yes / ☐ No
Non-English speaking   ☐ Yes / ☐ No

Hearing deficit   ☐ Yes / ☐ No
Sight deficit   ☐ Yes / ☐ No

Comments _____

Write out the entire doctor's order

☐ Cardiac US _____

☐ Fetal US _____

☐ US of abd _____

☐ US of pelvis _____

☐ US of GB _____

☐ Write in order _____

HEALTH UNIT COORDINATOR
HEALTH UNIT COORDINATOR PROCEDURES

JMP Medical Center

Patient Label

Doctor ordering _____

Date to be done _____ ☐ Stat ☐ Routine ☐ ASAP

Today's date _____ Requested by _____

MAGNETIC RESONANCE IMAGING REQUISITION

Clinical indication _____

Transportation ☐ Portable ☐ Stretcher ☐ Wheelchair ☐ Ambulatory

O₂ ☐ Yes / ☐ No

IV ☐ Yes / ☐ No

Isolation ☐ Yes / ☐ No

Diabetic ☐ Yes / ☐ No

Seizure disorder ☐ Yes / ☐ No

Non-English speaking ☐ Yes / ☐ No

Hearing deficit ☐ Yes / ☐ No

Sight deficit ☐ Yes / ☐ No

Comments _____

Write out the entire doctor's order

☐ MRI of brain _____

☐ MRI of spine _____

☐ MRI shoulder _____

☐ MRI knee _____

☐ MRA (magnetic resonance angiography) _____

☐ Write in order _____

JMP Medical Center

HEALTH UNIT COORDINATOR
HEALTH UNIT COORDINATOR PROCEDURES

Doctor ordering _____

Date to be done _____ ☐ Stat ☐ Routine ☐ ASAP

Today's date _____ Requested by _____

Patient Label

NUCLEAR MEDICINE REQUISITION

Clinical indication _____

Transportation ☐ Portable ☐ Stretcher ☐ Wheelchair ☐ Ambulatory

O_2 ☐ Yes / ☐ No   Diabetic ☐ Yes / ☐ No   Hearing deficit ☐ Yes / ☐ No

IV ☐ Yes / ☐ No   Seizure disorder ☐ Yes / ☐ No   Sight deficit ☐ Yes / ☐ No

Isolation ☐ Yes / ☐ No   Non-English speaking ☐ Yes / ☐ No

Comments _____

Write out the entire doctor's order

☐ Adenosine / thallium scan _____

☐ Bone scan (total) _____

☐ Bone scan (regional) _____

☐ Breast scintigraphy _____

☐ Cardiac scan _____

☐ Liver and spleen _____

☐ Gallium scan _____

☐ GI bleeding scan _____

☐ Thyroid uptake and scan _____

☐ DISIDA _____

☐ Neutrospec scan _____

☐ PET _____

☐ MUGA _____

☐ Scrotal nuclear imaging _____

☐ Thallium stress scan _____

☐ Sestamibi stress _____

☐ WBC scan _____

☐ Vent/Perfus (VQ) _____

☐ Lung _____

☐ HIDA scan _____

☐ Write in order _____

JMP Medical Center

HEALTH UNIT COORDINATOR
HEALTH UNIT COORDINATOR PROCEDURES

Doctor ordering _____

Date to be done _____ ☐ Stat ☐ Routine ☐ ASAP

Today's date _____ Requested by _____

Patient Label

CARDIOVASCULAR DEPARTMENT REQUISITION

Clinical indication _____

Cardiac medications _____

Pacemaker? ☐ Yes / ☐ No   Type _____ Ht _____ Wt _____

Comments _____

LOC? ☐ Yes / ☐ No

Noninvasive Studies

☐ Arterial Stiffness Index

☐ Ankle Brachial Index

☐ Cardiac monitor

☐ Carotid Doppler flow analysis

☐ Chemical stress test

☐ Doppler flow studies _____

☐ Echocardiogram 2D M-Mode

☐ EKG / ECG / 12-lead

☐ Plethysmography _____

☐ EKG c̄ rhythm strip

☐ Holter monitor _____ hrs

☐ IPG

☐ Thallium stress test

☐ Sestamibi stress test

☐ Trans-esophageal echocardiogram

☐ Treadmill stress test

☐ Vascular duplex scan

☐ Vascular us

☐ Write in order _____

Invasive Studies

☐ Cardiac catheterization

☐ EPS

☐ Write in order _____

Transportation ☐ Portable ☐ Stretcher ☐ Wheelchair ☐ Ambulatory

O₂ ☐ Yes / ☐ No   Diabetic ☐ Yes / ☐ No   Hearing deficit ☐ Yes / ☐ No

IV ☐ Yes / ☐ No   Seizure disorder ☐ Yes / ☐ No   Sight deficit ☐ Yes / ☐ No

Isolation ☐ Yes / ☐ No   Non-English speaking ☐ Yes / ☐ No

HEALTH UNIT COORDINATOR
HEALTH UNIT COORDINATOR PROCEDURES

JMP Medical Center

Patient Label

Doctor ordering _____

Date to be done _____   ☐ Stat   ☐ Routine   ☐ ASAP

Today's date _____   Requested by _____

NEUROLOGY DEPARTMENT REQUISITION

Anticonvulsant medication _____

Clinical indication _____

Transportation   ☐ Portable   ☐ Stretcher   ☐ Wheelchair   ☐ Ambulatory

O₂   ☐ Yes / ☐ No
IV   ☐ Yes / ☐ No
Isolation ☐ Yes / ☐ No

Diabetic   ☐ Yes / ☐ No
Seizure disorder   ☐ Yes / ☐ No
Non-English speaking   ☐ Yes / ☐ No

Hearing deficit   ☐ Yes / ☐ No
Sight deficit   ☐ Yes / ☐ No

Comments _____

Write out the entire doctor's order _____

☐ Auditory Evoked Response (AER) _____

☐ BAER _____

☐ Caloric study _____

☐ EEG _____

☐ EMG _____

☐ ENG _____

☐ Nerve conduction studies _____

☐ SEP _____

☐ VER _____

☐ Write in order _____

JMP Medical Center

HEALTH UNIT COORDINATOR
HEALTH UNIT COORDINATOR PROCEDURES

Patient Label

Doctor ordering _____

Date to be done _____ Time to be done _____

Today's date _____ Requested by _____

ENDOSCOPY DEPARTMENT REQUISITION

Clinical indication _____

Transportation ☐ Portable ☐ Stretcher ☐ Wheelchair ☐ Ambulatory

O_2 ☐ Yes / ☐ No

IV ☐ Yes / ☐ No

Diabetic ☐ Yes / ☐ No Hearing deficit ☐ Yes / ☐ No

Seizure disorder ☐ Yes / ☐ No Sight deficit ☐ Yes / ☐ No

Isolation ☐ Yes / ☐ No Non-English speaking ☐ Yes / ☐ No

Pre-op medication ☐ Yes / ☐ No Time given _____

Comments _____

☐ Arthroscopy ☐ Esophagoscopy ☐ Pelvioscopy

☐ Bronchoscopy ☐ Fetoscopy ☐ Peritoneoscopy

☐ Colonoscopy ☐ Gastroscopy ☐ Proctoscopy

☐ Colposcopy ☐ Hysteroscopy ☐ Sigmoidoscopy

☐ Cystoscopy ☐ Laparoscopy ☐ Sinus endoscopy

☐ Enteroscopy ERCP ☐ Mediastinoscopy ☐ Thoracoscopy

☐ EGD ☐ Trans-esophageal echocardiogram (TEE)

☐ Write in order _____

HEALTH UNIT COORDINATOR
HEALTH UNIT COORDINATOR PROCEDURES

JMP Medical Center

Patient Label

Doctor ordering _____

Date to be done _____   ☐ Stat   ☐ Routine   ☐ ASAP

Today's date _____   Requested by _____

CARDIOPULMONARY (RESPIRATORY CARE) DEPARTMENT – DIAGNOSTICS REQUISITION

Clinical indication _____

Anticoagulant medication?   ☐ Yes   Name of medication _____
                             ☐ No

Room air   ☐ Yes / ☐ No   Oxygen ☐ Yes / ☐ No   If yes, _____ L/min

Comments _____

☐ ABG

☐ CBG   ☐ Pre-op teaching

☐ CPR Teaching   ☐ PFTs   ☐ Spirometry

☐ Pulse oximetry   ☐ with bronchodilators

☐ Write in order   ☐ without bronchodilators

HEALTH UNIT COORDINATOR
HEALTH UNIT COORDINATOR PROCEDURES

JMP Medical Center

Patient Label

Doctor ordering _____

Date to be done _____ ☐ Stat ☐ Routine ☐ ASAP

Today's date _____ Requested by _____

CARDIOPULMONARY (RESPIRATORY CARE) DEPARTMENT - TREATMENT REQUISITION

Clinical indication _____

Comments _____

☐ O₂ _____ L/M ☐ NP ☐ Mask ☐ Tent ☐ Other
☐ Aerosol delivery type _____
☐ Bi-level press. vent. _____
☐ BiPAP _____
☐ CPAP _____
☐ CPT _____
☐ IPPB _____
☐ IS _____
☐ SVN _____
☐ USN _____
☐ Write in order _____

Ventilator orders
IMV mode _____ TV _____ FIO₂ _____ PO₂ _____ PS _____ Peep

☐ Write in order _____

HEALTH UNIT COORDINATOR
HEALTH UNIT COORDINATOR PROCEDURES

JMP Medical Center

Patient Label

Doctor ordering _____

☐ Stat   ☐ Routine   ☐ ASAP

Today's date _____   Requested by _____

ORTHOPEDIC/TRACTION EQUIPMENT REQUISITION

Diagnosis _____

Comments _____

Write out the entire doctor's order

☐ Write in order _____

☐ Bryant's _____

☐ Bucks _____

☐ Cervical _____

☐ Overhead frame and trapeze _____

☐ Russell's _____

☐ Split Russell's _____

HEALTH UNIT COORDINATOR
HEALTH UNIT COORDINATOR PROCEDURES

JMP Medical Center

Patient Label

Doctor ordering _____

Today's date _____   Time to be done _____

Date to be done _____   Requested by _____

PHYSICAL THERAPY REQUISITION

Clinical indication

Transportation ☐ Portable ☐ Stretcher ☐ Wheelchair ☐ Ambulatory

O_2 ☐ Yes / ☐ No   Diabetic   ☐ Yes / ☐ No
IV   ☐ Yes / ☐ No   Seizure disorder   ☐ Yes / ☐ No
Isolation   ☐ Yes / ☐ No   Non-English speaking ☐ Yes / ☐ No

Hearing deficit ☐ Yes / ☐ No
Sight deficit   ☐ Yes / ☐ No

Comments _____

Write out the entire doctor's order _____

☐ CMP
☐ Crutch training
☐ ES
☐ Exercise orders
☐ Evaluation
☐ Hot packs
☐ Hubbard tank
☐ Hyperbaric oxygen tx
☐ ROM
☐ Shortwave diathermy
☐ TENs
☐ Ultrasound c̄ massage
☐ Walker training
☐ Whirlpool
☐ Write in order

HEALTH UNIT COORDINATOR
HEALTH UNIT COORDINATOR PROCEDURES

JMP Medical Center

Patient Label

Doctor ordering _____ Time to be done _____

Date to be done _____ Requested by _____

Today's date _____

OCCUPATIONAL THERAPY REQUISITION

Clinical indication

Transportation ☐ Portable ☐ Stretcher ☐ Wheelchair ☐ Ambulatory

O_2 ☐ Yes / ☐ No   Diabetic ☐ Yes / ☐ No   Hearing deficit ☐ Yes / ☐ No

IV ☐ Yes / ☐ No   Seizure disorder ☐ Yes / ☐ No   Sight deficit ☐ Yes / ☐ No

Isolation ☐ Yes / ☐ No   Non-English speaking ☐ Yes / ☐ No

Comments

Write out the entire doctor's order _____

☐ ADL _____

☐ Evaluation and treatment as needed

☐ Increase mobility

☐ Supply and train in adaptive equipment (e.g., Use ADL button hooks and feeding utensils)

☐ Write in order _____

APPENDIX C

The Clinical Evaluation Record

The main purpose of the clinical evaluation record is to measure and document the student's performance on the nursing unit. The clinical evaluation record is divided into seven units; the first six are sequenced according to the increasing degree of knowledge and skill the student needs to complete the unit. The objectives and corresponding activities will assist the student in mastering each of the skills required to complete the tasks. A rating scale of competent (C) or not competent (N) is provided to document the student's performance level.

The clinical evaluation record tells the student, the instructor, and the preceptor exactly what is expected of the student during his or her clinical experience. Use of this record allows the student to pursue mastery of skills and allows the instructor or preceptor to evaluate the student's skills. The completed form becomes a written record of the student's performance in the clinical setting. The form may be used by the instructor to determine grades, or by the student to obtain employment. As with the rest of this manual, this appendix corresponds with the textbook, *LaFleur Brooks' Health Unit Coordinating*, 7th edition.

To ensure overall competence of student performance, the following course requirements are recommended. To successfully complete the health unit coordinator clinical experience, the student must:

1. Perform the tasks listed in this appendix with a rating of C.
2. Have no more than _____ hour(s) of unexcused absences.
3. Behave in an ethical manner and not in any way jeopardize the safety or welfare of patients or co-workers.
4. Demonstrate the ability to form interpersonal relationships with other hospital employees, which is necessary for the delivery of quality patient care.
5. Accept feedback from the instructor and health care facility staff and make changes requested by the instructor.
6. Demonstrate the ability to function during stressful situations on the nursing unit.

Outline

To the Evaluator

The clinical evaluation record clearly outlines for the student the activities that must be completed or performed to master the objectives for each unit. The student should notify you when ready to be evaluated in performing a task. Performance should be documented on the rating scale as follows:

C indicates competency; ability to perform the activity with minimal or no assistance in a manner that would qualify the student for employment as a health unit coordinator in a health care facility.

N indicates that further practice is needed to demonstrate competency or that there is an inability to perform the task with minimal or no assistance in a manner that would qualify the student for employment as a health unit coordinator in a health care facility. Reasons for an *N* rating and activities to improve performance should be outlined to the student.

To use the clinical evaluation record to its full potential, we suggest that the student cross out procedural steps not used in their clinical setting and write in steps that are used but not included here. This is particularly important when the student is in a facility with electronic medical records that has implemented computer physician order entry. It may be useful to have the student compile an additional skills list to be submitted along with the clinical evaluation record.

To the Student

The clinical evaluation record contains objectives for many of the tasks that you must perform in order to complete the clinical course. Activities are included to assist you in completing the objectives. Some of the activities require you to answer questions in writing. After you have completed these activities, give them to your instructor for evaluation. If they are satisfactory, the instructor will circle *C* on the rating scale. If they are not satisfactory, the instructor will circle *N* on the rating scale. Other activities require your instructor or preceptor to observe your performance. You may practice these activities as often as necessary to achieve competency. When you are ready to have your performance evaluated, ask your instructor or preceptor to observe you while you perform the activity. If you perform the activity satisfactorily, the instructor will circle *C* on the rating scale. If your performance is less than satisfactory, your instructor will circle *N* on the rating scale. Reasons for an *N* rating and activities to improve performance will be outlined for you by your instructor.

The clinical evaluation record allows you to plan your clinical activities and to judge your own performance of health unit coordinator tasks. It also becomes a written record of your progress throughout the clinical experience. Become familiar with the entire form. The units are sequenced according to the increasing degree of skill required to perform the activity; however, you do not need to perform the activities in order of the units. Perform the activities for evaluation when you are ready and when the opportunity presents itself. The only requirement is that you complete the pertinent activities satisfactorily by the end of your clinical experience.

To use the clinical evaluation record to its full potential, we suggest that you cross out procedural steps not used in your clinical setting and write in steps that are used but not included here. If your clinical placement is in a facility with electronic medical records that has implemented computer physician order entry, you may be required to compile an additional skills list to be submitted along with the clinical evaluation record.

UNIT 1

INTRODUCTION TO THE HEALTH CARE FACILITY

The following activities are designed to help you meet the objectives for this unit. You will need to be evaluated by your preceptor or instructor as you perform each activity. Each activity should be completed with a *C* (competent) score by the end of the first week of the clinical session.

Objective 1: Locate the following on the nursing unit:

	Evaluation		Initials
Kitchen	C	N	_____
Clean utility room	C	N	_____
Dirty utility room	C	N	_____
Medication room	C	N	_____

Report room	C	N	_____
Central supply closet	C	N	_____
Linen closet	C	N	_____
Pneumatic tube	C	N	_____
Code cart	C	N	_____
Fire extinguisher	C	N	_____
Telephone code button or direct number	C	N	_____
Shredder (if applicable)	C	N	_____
Fax machine	C	N	_____
Printer	C	N	_____
Scanner (if applicable)	C	N	_____
Locator (if applicable)	C	N	_____
Admission packet	C	N	_____
Surgery packet	C	N	_____
Supplemental forms	C	N	_____

Objective 2: Write the names of the following health care personnel on the nursing unit.

Health unit coordinator _____

Nurse (clinical) manager _____

Team leader (if applicable) _____

Shift manager _____

Staff nurses _____

Patient care technicians _____

Certified nursing assistants _____

Other _____

Objective 3: Describe the duties of the health care personnel listed.

Health unit coordinator _____

Nurse (clinical) manager _____

Team leader (if applicable) _____

Shift manager _____

Staff nurses _____

Patient care technicians _____

Certified nursing assistants _____

Other _____

Objective 4: Write the name of the services provided by the nursing unit (for example, medical or pediatric).

_____   C   N   _____

Objective 5: Locate the following departments in the hospital.

Nursing administration office	C	N	_____
Staffing office	C	N	_____
Human resources	C	N	_____
Employee health	C	N	_____
Cafeteria	C	N	_____
Admitting department	C	N	_____
Case management department	C	N	_____
Health information systems or medical records department	C	N	_____
Pharmacy department	C	N	_____
Laboratory department	C	N	_____
Diagnostic imaging department	C	N	_____
Cardiopulmonary (respiratory care) department	C	N	_____
Neurology department	C	N	_____
Physical and occupational therapy departments	C	N	_____
Morgue	C	N	_____
Other _____	C	N	_____

Objective 6: Demonstrate the use of the pneumatic tube system for conveying devices by sending a tube or conveyor to another area of the hospital.

_____   C   N   _____

**Objective 7: Demonstrate the correct
assembly and labeling of a patient's
chart.**

_____   C   N   _____

**Objective 8: Locate the area where patient
care forms are stored.**

_____   C   N   _____

**Objective 9: Identify the standard forms
used to prepare a patient's chart at the
time of admission to the unit.**

_____   C   N   _____

**Objective 10: Collect a sample of the
following supplemental forms.**

Parenteral fluid record form   C   N   _____

Therapy record forms for various departments C   N   _____

Frequent vital signs record form   C   N   _____

Diabetic, anticoagulant, or other flow sheet C   N   _____

Surgical consent form   C   N   _____

Consent for blood transfusion   C   N   _____

**Objective 11: List other supplemental
forms used on the nursing unit.**

_____   C   N   _____

_____   C   N   _____

**Objective 12: a. Locate the area on the nursing unit where
the central service department supplies are stored.**

_____   C   N   _____

b. List 10 items stored on your unit (central supply floor stock).

1. _____   C   N   _____

2. _____   C   N   _____

3. _____   C   N   _____

4. _____   C   N   _____

5. _____   C   N   _____

6. _____   C   N   _____

7. _____   C   N   _____

8. _____   C   N   _____

9. _____   C   N   _____

10. _____   C   N   _____

Objective 13: Locate the following resource materials on the nursing unit (may be computerized or hard copy).

Physicians' Desk Reference and *Nursing Drug Handbook*	C	N	_____
Medical dictionary	C	N	_____
Policy and procedure manual	C	N	_____
Disaster manual	C	N	_____
Laboratory manual	C	N	_____
Diagnostic imaging manual	C	N	_____
Web site of the human resources department	C	N	_____
Other _____	C	N	_____

Objective 14: Locate the surgery schedule for your nursing unit and identify which patients from your floor are scheduled for surgery.

_____   C   N   _____

Performance Acceptable   ❑

Additional Practice and Reevaluation Needed   ❑

Recommendations to Improve Performance: _____

_____

_____

_____

Preceptor's Comments: _____

_____

_____

_____

Instructor's Comments: _____

_____

_____

_____

Student's Comments: _____

_____

_____

_____

UNIT 2

HEALTH UNIT COORDINATOR COMMUNICATION SKILLS AND PROFESSIONALISM

The following activities are designed to help you meet the objectives for this unit. You will need to be evaluated by your preceptor or instructor as you perform the activities. Each activity should be completed with a C (competent) score by the end of the clinical session.

Objective 1: Demonstrate communication skills.

	Evaluation		Initials
Communicate with patients, visitors, and staff in a professional and empathetic manner.	C	N	_____
Communicate admissions, discharges, and transfers to nursing staff and admitting department in a timely manner.	C	N	_____
Contact physicians, ancillary services, and other departments as requested.	C	N	_____
Use problem-solving techniques to resolve conflicts.	C	N	_____
Familiarize yourself with staff and staff assignments.	C	N	_____
Listen to the change-of-shift report and take notes as needed.	C	N	_____
Demonstrate sensitivity to cultural diversity.	C	N	_____
Respond to difficult situations using appropriate assertiveness.	C	N	_____
Demonstrate coping techniques in stressful situations.	C	N	_____

Objective 2: Demonstrate professional standards.

	Evaluation		Initials
Arrive prior to the beginning of your shift, prepared to work.	C	N	_____
If unable to attend your clinical session:	C	N	_____
Notify the nursing unit at least _____ hours prior to the start of assigned shift.	C	N	_____
Notify your instructor at least _____ hours prior to the start of assigned shift.	C	N	_____
Take assigned breaks without exceeding time; be at assigned station at all other times.	C	N	_____
Conform to the dress code outlined by hospital or school program.	C	N	_____
Follow guidelines for personal hygiene.	C	N	_____

Demonstrate respect for program and facility guidelines for cellphone use, smoking, and food consumption.   C   N   _____

Wear identification name tag.   C   N   _____

Demonstrate courtesy and professionalism at all times.   C   N   _____

Complete tasks accurately and in a timely manner.   C   N   _____

Use free time to enhance job performance by familiarizing yourself with unit and department manuals.   C   N   _____

Performance Acceptable   ❑

Additional Practice and Reevaluation Needed   ❑

Recommendations to Improve Performance: _____

_____

_____

_____

Preceptor's Comments: _____

_____

_____

_____

Instructor's Comments: _____

_____

_____

_____

Student's Comments: _____

_____

_____

_____

UNIT 3

COMMUNICATION DEVICES

The following activities are designed to help you meet the objectives for this unit. You will need to be evaluated by your preceptor or instructor as you perform the activities. Each activity should be completed with a C (competent) score by the end of the clinical session.

Objective 1: Demonstrate effective telephone communication skills when answering incoming calls.

	Evaluation		Initials
Answer the telephone as quickly as possible.	C	N	_____
Excuse yourself, if necessary, from discussions within the nursing unit prior to answering the telephone.	C	N	_____
Identify the nursing unit, your name, and your title.	C	N	_____
Have a pencil and paper at hand to write pertinent information.	C	N	_____
Speak clearly and distinctly and use a pleasant tone.	C	N	_____
Ask pertinent questions to establish the caller's identity.	C	N	_____
Refer all calls regarding a patient's care, status, and so forth to the preceptor or nurse.	C	N	_____
Communicate the caller's name, the nature of the call, and the telephone number to the person to whom the call is being referred.	C	N	_____
Put the caller on hold correctly when needed.	C	N	_____
Successfully transfer the caller as needed.	C	N	_____
Accurately record laboratory or other diagnostic results with appropriate notification of health care personnel regarding critical values	C	N	_____

Objective 2: Demonstrate effective telephone communication skills when making outgoing calls.

Plan the conversation prior to making the call by gathering all of the pertinent information.	C	N	_____
Identify yourself to the person receiving the call by naming the hospital, the nursing unit, and your name and title.	C	N	_____

Objective 3: Demonstrate effective telephone communication skills when leaving a voice mail message.

Speak slowly and distinctly.	C	N	_____
If the message includes a name, give the first and last name and spell the last name.	C	N	_____

If the message includes a telephone number, repeat the number at the beginning and at the end of the message.   C   N   _____

Objective 4: Demonstrate effective telephone communication skills when paging.

Demonstrate the use of a digital pager by paging your instructor.   C   N   _____

Page hospital personnel as requested to do so.   C   N   _____

Objective 5: Demonstrate the use of fax machine by faxing pharmacy copies.

_____   C   N   _____

Objective 6: Demonstrate the use of scanner by scanning standard chart forms.

_____   C   N   _____

Objective 7: Demonstrate appropriate communication skills using the intercom.

Demonstrate use of the intercom to initiate and receive calls, speaking with appropriate volume.   C   N   _____

Use discretion when transmitting information via the intercom to avoid patients' embarrassment or alarm and the disclosure of confidential information.   C   N   _____

Objective 8: Demonstrate the use of locator or wireless device by locating hospital personnel.

_____   C   N   _____

Objective 9: Demonstrate required computer skills.

Sign on to the computer using assigned code.   C   N   _____

Sign off the computer when leaving the nursing unit.   C   N   _____

Demonstrate appropriate use of e-mail.   C   N   _____

Locate doctor's name and telephone number from computerized doctors' roster.   C   N   _____

Locate a patient on another unit by name.   C   N   _____

Locate all pending orders on a patient on your unit.   C   N   _____

Locate laboratory results on a patient on your unit.   C   N   _____

Order supplies from the supply purchasing department.   C   N   _____

Print a census for your unit.   C   N   _____

Print patient labels and a face or information sheet for your unit.   C   N   _____

Enter demographic information for a newly admitted patient.   C   N   _____

Performance Acceptable   ❑

Additional Practice and Reevaluation Needed   ❑

Recommendations to Improve Performance: _____

_____

_____

_____

Preceptor's Comments: _____

_____

_____

_____

Instructor's Comments: _____

_____

_____

_____

Student's Comments: _____

_____

_____

_____

UNIT 4

LEGALITIES AND CONFIDENTIALITY: DEALING WITH PATIENT INFORMATION

The following activities are designed to help you meet the objectives for this unit. You will need to be evaluated by your preceptor or instructor as you perform the activities. Each activity should be completed with a *C* (competent) score by the end of the clinical session.

Objective 1: Demonstrate knowledge and application of the Health Insurance Portability and Accountability Act requirements.

	Evaluation		Initials
Discuss patient information only when required to do so for patient care purposes and in the confines of the nursing unit.	C	N	_____
Allow access to patient charts to authorized health care personnel only.	C	N	_____
Copy patient chart forms only when requested to do so in a doctor's order and only after checking and following the hospital policy on copying patient chart forms.	C	N	_____
Provide information only when instructed to do so by authorized nursing personnel.	C	N	_____

Objective 2: Demonstrate the following legal guidelines when dealing with patient charts and legal documents.

Write accurately and legibly when preparing a surgical consent.	C	N	_____
Do not obliterate or white-out information on a legal document.	C	N	_____
Performance Acceptable	❏		
Additional Practice and Reevaluation Needed	❏		

Recommendations to Improve Performance: _____

_____

_____

_____

Preceptor's Comments: _____

_____

_____

_____

Instructor's Comments: _____

_____

_____

_____

Student's Comments: _____

_____

_____

_____

UNIT 5

ROUTINE HEALTH UNIT COORDINATOR TASKS

The following activities are designed to help you meet the objectives for this unit. The objectives of this unit are "performance objectives." You will be evaluated by your instructor or preceptor as you perform the activities. Each activity should be completed with a *C* score by the end of the clinical experience.

Objective 1: Given a written set of 20 or more vital signs, graph the temperature, pulse, and respiration (TPR) and blood pressure (BP) on patients' graphic sheets.

	Evaluation		**Initials**
_____	C	N	_____

Objective 2: Order daily diagnostic tests for the patients on your unit.

_____	•C	N	_____

Objective 3: Transcribe admission, transfer, and discharge data on the daily census record.

_____	C	N	_____

Objective 4: File diagnostic reports in patients' charts. Compare each patient's name on the diagnostic report with the patient's name on the back of the chart.

_____	C	N	_____

Performance Acceptable ❏

Additional Practice and Reevaluation Needed ❏

Recommendations to Improve Performance: _____

_____

_____

_____

Preceptor's Comments: _____

_____

_____

_____

Instructor's Comments: _____

_____

_____

_____

Student's Comments: _____

_____

_____

_____

UNIT 6

TRANSCRIPTION OF PHYSICIANS' ORDERS

The following activities are designed to help you meet the objectives for this unit. You will need to be evaluated by your preceptor or instructor as you perform the activities. Each activity should be completed with a *C* (competent) score by the end of the clinical session.

Objective 1: Transcribe activity, positioning, and nursing observation orders.

	Evaluation		Initials
Bathroom privileges (BRP)	C	N	_____
Absolute bedrest (ABR)	C	N	_____
Head of bed elevated thirty degrees (HOB ≠ 30°)	C	N	_____
Intake and output (I & O)	C	N	_____
Vital signs order (VS)	C	N	_____
Pulse oximetry	C	N	_____
Bladder scanner	C	N	_____
Other _____	C	N	_____

Objective 2: Transcribe nursing treatment orders.

Catheterization order	C	N	_____
Enema order	C	N	_____
Blood transfusion order	C	N	_____
Other _____	C	N	_____

Objective 3: Transcribe nutritional care orders.

Regular diet	C	N	_____
Consistency (soft, clear liquid, full liquid) diet	C	N	_____
Therapeutic (American Diabetic Association [ADA], cardiac, renal) diet	C	N	_____
Total parenteral nutrition (TPN)	C	N	_____
Other _____	C	N	_____

Objective 4: Transcribe medication orders.

Type

Antiinfective	C	N	_____
Narcotic	C	N	_____
Hypnotic	C	N	_____
Antiarrhythmic	C	N	_____
Anticoagulant	C	N	_____
Other _____	C	N	_____

Frequency

Whenever necessary (prn)	C	N	_____
Daily (qd)	C	N	_____
Standing (bid, tid, quid, q _____ h)	C	N	_____
Immediately (stat)	C	N	_____
Notifcation of nurse or pharmacist for stat	C	N	_____
One time only	C	N	_____
Discontinue medication order (DC)	C	N	_____
Change in medication order	C	N	_____
Renewal of medication order	C	N	_____

Objective 5: Transcribe laboratory orders.

Hematology

Complete blood cell count (CBC)	C	N	_____
Prothrombin time (PT)	C	N	_____
Hemoglobin and hematocrit (H & H)	C	N	_____
Other _____	C	N	_____

Chemistry

Electrolytes (lytes)	C	N	_____
Comprehensive metabolic panel (CMP)	C	N	_____
Basic metabolic panel (BMP)	C	N	_____
Fasting blood sugar (FBS)	C	N	_____
Two-hour postprandial blood sugar (2-hr PP BS)	C	N	_____
Medication peak and trough	C	N	_____
Other _____	C	N	_____

Microbiology

Blood cultures	C	N	_____
Stool for *Clostridium difficile* (*C. diff*)	C	N	_____
Urine culture and sensitivity (C & S)	C	N	_____
Sputum for acid-fast bacilli (AFB)	C	N	_____
Other _____	C	N	_____

Serology

Human immunodeficiency virus screen ($HIVB_{24}AG$)	C	N	_____
Carcinoembryonic antigen (CEA)	C	N	_____
Rheumatoid factor	C	N	_____
Other _____	C	N	_____

Blood Bank

Type and crossmatch (T & x-match)	C	N	_____
Packed cells (PC)	C	N	_____
Platelets (plts or plt ct)	C	N	_____
Coombs test	C	N	_____
Other _____	C	N	_____

Cytology

Papanicolaou (pap) smear	C	N	_____
Other _____	C	N	_____

Other Specimens

Urine (UA)	C	N	_____
Cerebrospinal fluid (CSF)	C	N	_____
Bone marrow biopsy	C	N	_____
Pleural fluid	C	N	_____
Other _____	C	N	_____

Point of Care Testing (POCT)

Blood glucose monitoring	C	N	_____
Electrolytes	C	N	_____
Hemoglobin/Hematocrit	C	N	_____
D-Dimer (coagulation testing)	C	N	_____
Arterial blood gases	C	N	_____
Guaiac all stools	C	N	_____
Other _____	C	N	_____

Objective 6: Transcribe diagnostic imaging orders.

Radiology Orders that Require Preparation

Upper gastrointestinal (UGI)	C	N	_____
Barium enema (BE)	C	N	_____
Intravenous urogram or pyelogram (IVU or IVP)	C	N	_____

Radiology Orders that do not Require a Preparation

Chest PA & Lat	C	N	_____
Kidney, ureters, and bladder (KUB)	C	N	_____
Skeletal x-ray	C	N	_____
Other _____	C	N	_____

Special Procedures

Angiogram, venogram, or arteriogram	C	N	_____
Other _____	C	N	_____

Computed Tomography (CT)

CT of brain or abdomen	C	N
Other _____	C	N

Magnetic Resonance Imaging (MRI)

MRI of spine, brain or abdomen	C	N
Other _____	C	N

Nuclear Medicine

Bone scan	C	N
Body scan (brain, liver, spleen)	C	N
Thyroid uptake scan	C	N
Stress test using dipyridamole/thallium, etc.	C	N
Other _____	C	N

Ultrasound (US)

Pelvic US	C	N
Other _____	C	N

Objective 7: Transcribe cardiopulmonary (respiratory care) orders.

Diagnostic Orders

Arterial blood gases (ABG)	C	N
Capillary blood gases (CBG)	C	N
Spirometry	C	N

Treatment Orders

Incentive spirometry	C	N
Small volume nebulizer (SVN)	C	N
Intermittent positive pressure breathing (IPPB)	C	N
Oxygen (O_2)	C	N
Other _____	C	N

Objective 8: Transcribe cardiovascular diagnostic orders.

Electrocardiogram (EKG or ECG)	C	N
Two-dimensional M-mode echocardiogram	C	N

Stress test   C   N   _____

Other _____   C   N   _____

Objective 9: Transcribe cardiac catheterization orders.

Percutaneous transluminal coronary angioplasty (PTCA)   C   N   _____

Pacemaker or intracardiac defibrillator (ICD) insertion   C   N   _____

Other _____   C   N   _____

Objective 10: Transcribe neurology orders.

Electroencephalogram (EEG)   C   N   _____

Electromyogram (EMG)   C   N   _____

Brainstem auditory evoked response (BAER)   C   N   _____

Other _____   C   N   _____

Objective 11: Transcribe physical therapy orders.

Whirlpool   C   N   _____

Crutch training   C   N   _____

Exercises   C   N   _____

Hot packs   C   N   _____

Other _____   C   N   _____

Objective 12: Transcribe occupational therapy orders.

Activities of daily living (ADL) evaluation   C   N   _____

Other _____   C   N   _____

Objective 13: Transcribe miscellaneous orders.

Case management   C   N   _____

Social services   C   N   _____

Consultation   C   N   _____

Wound management/hyperbaric medicine   C   N   _____

Other _____   C   N   _____

Performance Acceptable ❏

Additional Practice and Reevaluation Needed ❏

Recommendations to Improve Performance: _____

_____

_____

_____

Preceptor's Comments: _____

_____

_____

_____

Instructor's Comments: _____

_____

_____

_____

Student's Comments: _____

_____

_____

_____

UNIT 7

HEALTH UNIT COORDINATING PROCEDURES

The following activities are designed to help you meet the objectives for this unit. You will need to be evaluated by your preceptor or instructor as you perform the activities. Each activity should be completed with a *C* (competent) score by the end of the clinical session.

Objective 1: Perform admission procedures.	**Evaluation**		**Initials**
Greet the patient upon arrival at the nurse's station.	C	N	_____
Inform the patient that the nurse will be notified of his or her arrival.	C	N	_____
Notify the attending physician, hospital resident, or hospitalist of the patient's admission, and obtain orders.	C	N	_____
Move the patient's name from the admission screen on the computer to the correct bed in the nursing unit.	C	N	_____

Document the patient's admission on the admission, discharge, and transfer sheet and on the census or assignment board or sheet.	C N	_____
Check the patient's signature on the admission service agreement form (C of A).	C N	_____

Complete the procedure for the preparation of the chart:

a. Label all the chart forms with the patient's identification labels.	C N	_____
b. Fill in all the needed headings.	C N	_____
c. Place all the forms in the chart behind the proper dividers.	C N	_____
d. Label the outside of the chart.	C N	_____
Prepare any other labels or identification cards used by your facility.	C N	_____
Prepare any other patient files used by your facility.	C N	_____
Place the patient identification labels in the correct place in the patient's chart.	C N	_____
Document all the necessary information on the patient's Kardex form or in the computer if the Kardex form is computerized.	C N	_____
Place the Kardex form in the proper place in the Kardex holder.	C N	_____
Enter appropriate data into the computer patient profile screen.	C N	_____
Transcribe the data from the admission nurse's notes on the graphic sheet.	C N	_____
Document allergy information in all the designated areas.	C N	_____
Prepare an allergy bracelet with allergies written on it to be placed on the patient's wrist, if necessary.	C N	_____
Note code status on front of chart according to hospital guidelines, if necessary.	C N	_____
Place red tape stating "name alert" on spine of chart if there is another patient on the unit with the same or a similar name.	C N	_____
Add the patient's name to the required unit forms.	C N	_____
Transcribe the admission orders according to your hospital's policy.	C N	_____

Objective 2: Perform discharge procedures.

Read the entire order when transcribing the discharge order.	C N	_____
Check for any prescription that may have been left in chart by doctor.	C N	_____
Prepare patient discharge file if used by your facility.	C N	_____
Notify the nurse caring for the patient of the discharge order.	C N	_____
Notify bed placement or other appropriate departments.	C N	_____
Enter the status of "pending discharge" with expected departure time into the computer.	C N	_____

Explain the procedure for discharge to the patient and the patient's relatives.	C	N	_____
Notify other departments that were giving the patient daily treatments.	C	N	_____
Communicate the patient's discharge to the nutritional care department via computer.	C	N	_____
Arrange for clinic or other appointments if doctor requests it.	C	N	_____
Prepare credit slips for medications returned to the pharmacy or equipment and supplies from CSD.	C	N	_____
Notify nursing personnel or transportation service to transport patient to the discharge area.	C	N	_____
Write the patient's name on the admission, discharge, and transfer sheet.	C	N	_____
Delete the patient's name from the unit census or assignment board or sheet and TPR sheet.	C	N	_____
Notify environmental services to clean the discharged patient's room.	C	N	_____
Prepare the chart for the health information management department.	C	N	_____
Check the summary and DRG worksheet for the physician's summation and the patient's final diagnosis.	C	N	_____
Check for the correct patient identification labels on chart forms.	C	N	_____
Shred all chart forms that have been labeled and do not have any documentation on them.	C	N	_____
Check for "old records" or "split chart." Place the split chart in the proper sequence.	C	N	_____
Rearrange the chart forms in discharge sequence per your hospital policy.	C	N	_____
Send the chart of the discharged patient to the health information systems department along with old records of the patient.	C	N	_____
Prepare and print patient medication information and other educational materials to be given to patient.	C	N	_____
Prepare and print patient referrals if used by your facility.	C	N	_____
Discharge patient from computer after the patient leaves the unit.	C	N	_____
Make follow up calls to discharged patient regarding appointments and medication refills.	C	N	_____

Objective 3: Perform additional steps for discharge to another facility.

Notify case management or social service of the physician's orders to discharge to another facility. Transportation will usually be arranged by the case manager or social worker.	C	N	_____
Complete the continuing care form or transfer form (top section).	C	N	_____
Photocopy or print forms as necessary (follow hospital policy for procedure).	C	N	_____

Distribute continuing care form and copies as required (place a copy of continuing care form and chart copies in envelope to send with patient).   C   N   _____

Perform routine discharge steps.   C   N   _____

Objective 4: Perform additional steps for discharge home with assistance.

Notify case management or social service.   C   N   _____

Prepare the continuing care form.   C   N   _____

Obtain a release of information from patient.   C   N   _____

Photocopy or print forms as necessary (follow hospital policy for procedure).   C   N   _____

Distribute continuing care form and copies as required.   C   N   _____

Perform routine discharge steps.   C   N   _____

Objective 5: Perform postmortem procedures.

Contact the attending physician, staff physician, or resident when asked by nurse to verify the patient's death.   C   N   _____

Notify the hospital operator of patient's death according to hospital policy.   C   N   _____

Prepare any forms that may be needed.   C   N   _____

Notify the mortuary that was designated by the family (if requested to do so).   C   N   _____

Call the morgue if the body is to be taken for autopsy or is to remain there until mortuary personnel arrives.   C   N   _____

The nurse will gather the deceased's clothing and place it in a paper sack; you may be asked to label it with the patient's name, room number, and the date.   C   N   _____

Obtain the mortuary book from the nursing office or have a mortuary form prepared for the mortuary personnel.   C   N   _____

Notify all doctors who were involved with the patient's care.   C   N   _____

Perform routine discharge steps.   C   N   _____

Objective 6: Perform procedures for transfer of patient to another unit within the hospital.

Transcribe order for a transfer.   C   N   _____

Notify the patient's nurse of the transfer order.   C   N   _____

Notify admitting department of transfer order to get a room assignment.   C   N   _____

Communicate to the patient's nurse the receiving unit and room number as given by the admitting department.   C   N   _____

Notify the receiving unit of the transfer.   C   N   _____

Document the transfer on the unit admission, discharge, and transfer sheet.   C   N   _____

Immediately prior to the transfer of the patient, remove the chart forms from the chart holder and the Kardex form from the Kardex holder and obtain any medication administration records not filed in the chart.   C   N   _____

Erase the patient's name on the census or assignment board or sheet.   C   N   _____

Notify all departments that perform scheduled treatments on the patient.   C   N   _____

Indicate the transfer on the computer diet screen and on the TPR sheet.   C   N   _____

Notify the attending physician, all other physicians involved with the patient's care, the switchboard, information desk, the flower desk, and the mail room of the transfer.   C   N   _____

Follow procedures for discharge.   C   N   _____

Objective 7: Perform procedures for transfer of patient to another room on the same unit.

Transcribe order for a transfer.   C   N   _____

Notify the patient's nurse when the request for transfer is granted.   C   N   _____

Remove patient's chart from chart holder and place it in chart holder labeled with the new room number after printing corrected ID labels.   C   N   _____

Place all Kardex forms in their new places in the Kardex form holder.   C   N   _____

Move patient's name to the correct bed on computer census screen.   C   N   _____

Send change by computer to the nutritional care department and write the new room number on the TPR sheet.   C   N   _____

Document the transfer on the unit admission, discharge, and transfer sheet and on the census board.   C   N   _____

Notify environmental services to clean the room.   C   N   _____

Notify the switchboard and the information center of the change.   C   N   _____

Objective 8: Perform procedures for receiving a transferred patient.

Notify the nurse who will care for the patient of the expected arrival of a transferred patient.   C   N   _____

Introduce yourself to the transferred patient upon their arrival to the nursing unit.   C   N   _____

Notify the nurse of the transferred patient's arrival.   C   N   _____

Place the patient's chart in the correct chart holder.   C   N   _____

Print corrected patient ID labels and label patient's chart.   C   N   _____

Place allergy label on front of chart if necessary.	C N	_____
Place all Kardex forms in their proper places.	C N	_____
Note the receipt of a transferred patient on the unit admission, discharge, and transfer sheet, and write the patient's name on the census and assignment board or sheet.	C N	_____
Place the patient's name on the TPR sheet.	C N	_____
Move the patient's name from the previous unit and indicate the correct bed on the computer census screen.	C N	_____
Transcribe any new doctors' orders.	C N	_____

Objective 9: Perform preoperative procedures.

Label the surgery forms with the patient's identification labels and place them in the patient's chart.	C N	_____
Check the patient's chart for history and physical report.	C N	_____
Check the patient's chart for the following signed consent forms:		
Surgical consent.	C N	_____
Blood transfusion consent or refusal form.	C N	_____
Admission service agreement (C of A).	C N	_____
Check the patient's chart for any previously ordered studies such as labs and x-ray examinations.	C N	_____
Chart the patient's latest vital signs.	C N	_____
File the current medication administration record in the patient's chart.	C N	_____
Print at least five face sheets to place in chart.	C N	_____
Place at least three sheets of patient identification labels in the patient's chart.	C N	_____
Notify the appropriate nursing personnel when surgery calls for the patient.	C N	_____

Objective 10: Perform postoperative procedures

Inform the patient's nurse of the patient's arrival in the PACU.	C N	_____
Inform the patient's nurse of the expected arrival of the patient from the recovery room.	C N	_____
Place all operating records behind the proper divider.	C N	_____
Write the date of surgery and the surgical procedure in the designated place on the patient's Kardex form or in the computer.	C N	_____
Write the date of the surgery on the patient's graphic sheet.	C N	_____

Transcribe the physician's postoperative orders. Notify the appropriate departments and the patient's nurse of physician's stat orders.   C   N   _____

Performance Acceptable   ❑

Additional Practice and Reevaluation Needed   ❑

Recommendations to Improve Performance: _____

_____

_____

_____

Preceptor's Comments: _____

_____

_____

_____

Instructor's Comments: _____

_____

_____

_____

Student's Comments: _____

_____

_____

_____

UNIT 8

MANAGEMENT OF THE UNIT

The following activities are designed to help you meet the objectives for this unit. The objectives of this unit are "performance objectives." You will be evaluated by your instructor or preceptor as you perform the activities. Each activity should be completed with a *C* score by the end of the clinical experience.

Objective 1: Assign cell phones or wireless devices to unit staff with appropriate documentation.

                                              Evaluation   **Initials**

_____   C   N   _____

Objective 2: Add or remove nursing staff assignments to or from the treatment team, or assist with staffing assignments.

_____   C   N   _____

Objective 3: Monitor and maintain the electronic record.

_____   C   N   _____

Objective 4: Maintain inventories and order or request supplies, services, and equipment as directed, including office supplies, patient educational material, isolation and code carts.

_____   C   N   _____

Objective 5: Gather data and complete administrative reports (daily, weekly, monthly).

_____   C   N   _____

Objective 6: Coordinate and attend staff education events and inservices.

_____   C   N   _____

Objective 7: Assist with the management and capture of patient charges as necessary.

_____   C   N   _____

Performance Acceptable   ❏

Additional Practice and Reevaluation Needed   ❏

Recommendations to Improve Performance: _____

_____

_____

_____

_____

Preceptor's Comments: _____

_____

_____

_____

Instructor's Comments: _____

_____

_____

_____

Student's Comments: _____

_____

_____

_____

UNIT 9

ORGANIZATION AND PRIORITIZING SKILLS

The following activities are designed to help you meet the objectives for this unit. You will need to be evaluated by your preceptor or instructor as you perform the activities. Each activity should be completed with a *C* (competent) score by the end of the clinical session.

Objective 1: Demonstrate knowledge of code procedures.

	Evaluation		Initials
Demonstrate how you would call a code arrest when requested to do so.	C	N	_____
Demonstrate how you would respond to a fire drill when requested to do so.	C	N	_____
Describe your role in case of a disaster code as outlined in the hospital disaster manual.	C	N	_____

Objective 2: Perform tasks in a conscientious manner.

Upon completion of transcription of a set of doctor's orders, ask your preceptor or instructor to evaluate your correct use of symbols.	C	N	_____
Take laboratory test results over the phone. Write the patient's name, room number, the laboratory values, the date, the time, and the caller's name. Read this information back to the caller to verify accuracy.	C	N	_____
When taking a telephone call, write all information to be given to another person.	C	N	_____

Objective 3: Demonstrate accuracy when transcribing doctors' orders.

Before taking transcribed orders to your preceptor for evaluation, check yourself on each of the following. Did you:

Read all of the orders?	C	N	_____
Fax the pharmacy copies?	C	N	_____
Check for stats?	C	N	_____
Notify appropriate persons or departments of stat orders?	C	N	_____
Place telephone calls, if necessary?	C	N	_____
Order everything required?	C	N	_____

Document all of the orders on the Kardex forms?   C   N   _____

Communicate the necessary orders to the nursing staff?   C   N   _____

Use correct symbols?   C   N   _____

Sign off the completed orders?   C   N   _____

Objective 4: Demonstrate initiative.

Participate in planning daily activities with your preceptor.   C   N   _____

Express desire to master new and varied skills.   C   N   _____

Answer the telephone as quickly as possible.   C   N   _____

Use resource material to assist in obtaining needed information.   C   N   _____

Continue working, ask how you can help others, or use free time to enhance
job performance and knowledge, even when your preceptor is not on the unit.   C   N   _____

Take notes so that you can remember what you learned.   C   N   _____

Objective 5: Demonstrate thoroughness.

Check all charts for new doctors' orders before returning charts to the chart rack.   C   N   _____

Determine the most appropriate person to whom a phone message is to be
given, rather than giving it to the first possible person.   C   N   _____

Keep a personal record of unfinished tasks you intend to complete as soon
as possible.   C   N   _____

Objective 6: Demonstrate ability to establish priorities on the job.

You have returned to the nursing unit from a break. There are several charts in
the rack that are flagged to indicate new doctors' orders. Describe how you
would proceed with this situation.   C   N   _____

Explain why you should answer a ringing phone before responding to a verbal
request if they occur simultaneously, unless it is an emergency situation.   C   N   _____

Explain why a request to take a patient to surgery has more urgency than a
request to take a patient to radiology.   C   N   _____

Explain why it is sound management to check the charts of the patients
scheduled for surgery that day when you first arrive for duty on the nursing unit.   C   N   _____

Objective 7: Demonstrate ability to multitask.

Handle being interrupted by telephone calls while transcribing doctors' orders.   C   N   _____

Complete routine tasks when you have interruptions, such as the need to
assist visitors, doctors, nurses, and others.   C   N   _____

**Objective 8: Demonstrate the ability to
plan a day's activities.**

1. List the daily routine tasks you are now performing as part of your
   responsibilities in the nursing unit.   C   N   _____
   Health Unit Coordinator Tasks

   _____

   _____

   _____

   _____

   _____

   _____

   _____

2. Using your task list, plan your work routine for one day.   C   N   _____
   Time Health Unit Coordinator Tasks

   _____

   _____

   _____

   _____

   _____

   _____

   _____

   _____

3. Implement your work schedule plan. Make adjustments as necessary.
   Critique your plan.   C   N   _____
   a. What were the strengths in your plan?

   _____

   _____

   b. What were the weaknesses in your plan?

   _____

   _____

c. What changes will you make?

_____

_____

Performance Acceptable ☐

Additional Practice and Reevaluation Needed ☐

Recommendations to Improve Performance: _____

_____

_____

_____

Preceptor's Comments: _____

_____

_____

_____

Instructor's Comments: _____

_____

_____

_____

Student's Comments: _____

_____

_____

_____